'Through poetry, lush visual imagery, fascinating case histories and crystal clear explanations and point locations, John Kirkwood brings the body, soul and spirit of Five Element acupuncture to life. A labour of love and devotion, this is a book clinicians, students and patients of traditional Chinese medicine have long been waiting for. I will use it in all my teaching and will cherish my copy for years to come.'

– *Lorie Eve Dechar, author of* Five Spirits: Alchemical Acupuncture for Psychological and Spiritual Healing

'*The Way of the Five Elements* is an original and immensely practical addition to the growing literature of Five Element medicine. In addition to his lively descriptions of each element, John Kirkwood offers something new: explorations of individual acupoints that highlight their elemental qualities. In choosing a small handful of powerful points for each element, Kirkwood offers readers a highly accessible way into the very complex system of acupuncture points. Novice readers and journeyman practitioners alike will find insights and ideas for acupressure treatment of themselves and their clients.'

– *Gail Reichstein Rex, acupuncturist and author of* Wood Becomes Water: Chinese Medicine in Everyday Life *and* Earth Acupuncture: Healing the Living Landscape

The Way of the Five Elements

by the same author

The Way of the Five Seasons
Living with the Five Elements for Physical,
Emotional, and Spiritual Harmony
John Kirkwood
ISBN 978 1 84819 301 7
eISBN 9780 85701 252 4

of related interest

Keepers of the Soul
The Five Guardian Elements of Acupuncture
Nora Franglen
ISBN 978 1 84819 185 3
eISBN 978 0 85701 146 6

The 12 Chinese Animals
Create Harmony in your Daily Life
through Ancient Chinese Wisdom
Master Zhongxian Wu
ISBN 978 1 84819 031 3
eISBN 978 0 85701 015 5

The Way
of the
Five Elements

52 weeks of powerful acupoints for
physical, emotional, and spiritual health

JOHN KIRKWOOD

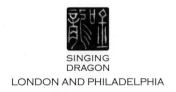

SINGING
DRAGON
LONDON AND PHILADELPHIA

First published in hardback in 2016
This edition published in 2018
by Singing Dragon
an imprint of Jessica Kingsley Publishers
73 Collier Street
London N1 9BE, UK
and
400 Market Street, Suite 400
Philadelphia, PA 19106, USA

www.singingdragon.com

Copyright © John Kirkwood 2016, 2018

Library of Congress Cataloging in Publication Data
A CIP catalog record for this book is available from the Library of Congress

British Library Cataloguing in Publication Data
A CIP catalogue record for this book is available from the British Library

ISBN 978 1 84819 414 4
eISBN 978 0 85701 216 6

Printed and bound in China

Contents

水

Notes on the Text

Throughout I have capitalised Element, Five Elements, Constitutional Element, Extraordinary Vessel, and the substances of Qi, Blood and Essence in order to distinguish from the more common usages of these words.

I have italicised Chinese words such as *shen* and *jing* but not Qi, yin or yang, which have more fully entered modern usage.

Preface

In 1991 I was very fortunate to study with Bob Duggan, Diane Connelly, Julia Measures and John Sullivan, teachers of the Traditional Acupuncture Institute (TAI) who were presenting their SOPHIA program in San Francisco. This year-long training, in five parts, introduced me to the sophisticated model of the Five Elements and to ways in which this perspective can be utilised in everyday life to bring health and balance.

I discovered that these Elements are not constituent parts like chemical components, but rather they are five unique vibrations that arise from the void, the Tao. Similar to the way light refracts into a spectrum of colours, the nature of the universe divides into distinct notes or vibrations. These vibrations pass through and inhabit all aspects of our material world. Everything resonates with these Elements.

One of the easiest ways to understand the Elements is through the qualities of the seasons which offer a direct experience of the nature of each Element. If we study the associations of an Element in its own season, there is an ambient energy that both highlights and supports the exploration.

I was so impressed with this model that I took it into my life and began to look at my own physical body, psyche, emotions and later my spiritual life from this perspective. Each year I delved more and more deeply into myself, learning through the Elements about my functioning, my strengths and struggles, where I am out of balance and where I am balanced.

After the SOPHIA program ended, a number of us who had completed the course decided to carry on meeting to continue the exploration. Out of this arose the whimsically named Five Hands Clapping group. We offered our own experiential workshops to the public and found that real healing was taking place in the participants, including ourselves. When the workshops finally ran their course, we continued to meet seasonally, setting up an environment that would echo the qualities of the season and the Element in order to understand more about ourselves through this work.

After I returned to Australia in 2006, I brought this perspective of living with the Elements into my acupressure classes, a quinterly newsletter, a blog and now this book. At each stage I have found that in order to bring the work to others I have, of necessity, plumbed my own depths to deeper and deeper levels. My physical health is better than it has been in the past, despite my advancing age; I am far more aware of and comfortable with my emotions; I have deep understandings about the connections between the different strands of my life; and I have come to know my true nature more fully and how this manifests uniquely in this location.

I hope that in this Five Element work you will find understanding, insight, inspiration, healing and balance. As I have.

Adelaide Hills
March 2015

Landscape of the Five Elements

This is a book that is meant not just to be read, but to be lived, explored, pondered and played with.

For the past 25 years, since I became closely acquainted with the Five Element model, I have been living my life as best I can by following the rhythms of nature, allowing them to teach me about myself. About my physical health, my preferences and dislikes, ideas and beliefs, emotions and even my spiritual journey. At the completion of each year, I come back to where I started in the seasonal cycle, but I am not the same person who started the year. I have changed at all levels, and the next cycle is altogether new. The work is not a repetition but a widening, deepening spiral of experience and understanding.

This book has been written from this perspective and invites you to learn from the Elements in their own seasons. Rather than read the book from start to finish, I suggest that you read this chapter, then begin with the chapter that relates to the Element of the season where you find yourself right now. If you are in winter, dive into the Water chapter; if it is spring in your neck of the woods, look at the Wood chapter; if summer is flourishing in your neighbourhood, check out Fire; if it is the late summer or harvest time for you, savour the delights of the Earth chapter; and if autumn is falling all around you, appreciate the gems that Metal has to offer.

There are a total of 52 entries, one for each week of the year. Each entry introduces an acupoint (sometimes two) and explores aspects of the Five Element model while providing information on how to use the point for your own health. Each Element chapter has ten or eleven entries that can be read, explored and lived with over the course of that season. You can treat the points on yourself or on others. Why not find a partner to trade with?

What I know from many years of doing this work is that when we explore the resonances, qualities and issues of an Element during its own season, the work goes deeper. For example, holding Water points in the winter will tend to have a greater effect than at other times of the year. Exploring your fear, the emotion of Water, will be more supported then. At the spiritual level, the truth that nothing is separate and that the Tao is the true nature of everything is more accessible in the darkest months of the year. The reason for this is that the energy of the Water Element is at its highest in winter and this ambient natural energy is available to support healing and growth in the Water realm.

Another way you might use the work is to consult the index for a particular condition you have and look at the acupoints that relate to that condition. But even using this symptomatic approach, you can consider the issues that relate to the points and their respective Elements in order to place your ailment in a wider, holistic context.

At one level you might use Gall Bladder 20 to relieve a headache. But you might also consider what is causing the headache. Is it that you are sitting under an air-conditioning draught at work and suffering from wind invasion? Perhaps you are angry and frustrated and the tension is concentrating at the back of your head. Maybe you didn't even realise you were angry. Possibly the headache stems from the fact that you can't see a clear path forward in your life because making plans and decisions is difficult for you. Going deeper still, you might ask yourself, 'What can I learn from this headache and how is it actually supporting my deepest unfolding?'

The Elements have so much to teach us. By paying attention to their lessons, particularly during their respective seasons when they are at their most potent, we have an opportunity to become more aware of ourselves, more fully who we are as human beings.

The Five Element model

Throughout this book I use the term Element to refer to the five different vibrations of all things. Some scholars and practitioners do not use the term Elements but refer to them as the five phases. This more accurately describes the cycle as a series of stages and avoids confusion with the concept of an element as a component part. While I agree that 'phase' is a more accurate description of what is occurring, I use the word Element because it has so thoroughly taken root in common usage. As long as it is clear that we are referring to a phase of a cycle and not to a constituent such as hydrogen, then I see no problem using the word Element.

Origins of the Five Elements

The earliest developments of the Five Element perspective are lost in the mists of Chinese prehistory, since writing did not develop in China until about 1200 BCE. But it is clear that this way of viewing the world was based on a close observation of nature. The perspective of the simple farmer who was in close contact with the rhythm of the seasons informed the development of the Five Element model.

The first articulation of this nature-based perspective was in the 3rd century BCE by the School of Naturalists, or the Yin-Yang school, which attempted to explain the universe in terms of the forces of nature: the polarity of yin (dark, cold, female, receptive) and yang (light, hot, male, assertive); and the Five Elements of Water, Wood, Fire, Earth and Metal. The perspectives of this early philosophical school became absorbed into the later development of Taoism.

The principles of the Naturalist school were laid out in the great classic, the *Neijing* or *The Yellow Emperor's Classic of Medicine*. The *Neijing* explains how the natural forces of yin and yang, Qi, and the Five Elements can be understood and used to bring balance and harmony to life. Thus, the *Neijing* not only gives details of a system of medicine, but is in fact a model of holistic living in all realms of human life. It does not separate external changes such as geographic, climatic and seasonal from internal changes such as emotions and reactions.[1] In this sense it is the first book of holistic medicine.

During the Qing dynasty of the Manchus (1644–1911) acupuncture began a long decline in favour of herbalism. What is more, the system utilised by herbalism was not related to the Five Element system, but to one known as Eight Principles for Differentiating Syndromes. Not only did acupuncture suffer a decline, but also one of the fundamental principles on which it had been founded, namely the Five Elements, lost its influence.

Another historical development contributed to the overall decline in all kinds of traditional medicine, namely that of rapid Westernisation in the latter part of the 19th century. Once Western allopathic medicine was introduced to China, it quickly supplanted the traditional medicine. This process was further accelerated by the collapse of the dynastic system in 1912. A law was passed in 1929 prohibiting the practice of the old medicine. The period that followed saw China descend into the chaos of civil war, invasion by Japan and further civil war, culminating in the eventual takeover by the Communists in 1949.

Taking over a ravaged country, Mao Tse-Tung was eager to find a system of health care that would support China's vast, growing and impoverished population, and so turned to the traditional methods. He encouraged the development of a new system of medicine based on traditional methods but which was in alignment with the Communist principles of rationalism and atheism. What emerged was a system that became known as traditional Chinese medicine (TCM), a system that became codified and taught in colleges rather than by the old way of learning from a master.[2]

Five Elements go West

Such was the system that was in place when Richard Nixon made his historic visit to China in 1972, an event that radically opened China to Western contact and trade. The form of acupuncture and herbalism that was subsequently exported to the West was a system that had been carefully culled of anything of a spiritual nature and which contained little of Five Element theory.

However, the ancient methods that predated the development of TCM were rescued and preserved by Europeans.[3] The French sinologist

Soulié Morant published works on acupuncture in French as early as 1929. His writings contain much that was to find its way into Five Element acupuncture but was omitted from TCM.

Another Frenchman, Jacques Lavier, was responsible for the spread of these ideas in Europe through his writings and the conferences he organised. Lavier exerted a particularly strong influence upon the early English acupuncturists and could be said to have been the principal cause of the early elevation of the Five Element method in England. English acupuncturists Denis Lawson-Wood,[4] Felix Mann[5] and Mary Austin[6] all published books on acupuncture which focused on this method.

It was in this climate that J.R. Worsley, an osteopath, began to study acupuncture. He attended Lavier's historic 1963 seminar in London and later made trips to China, Taiwan and Japan to study with masters whose techniques were largely in alignment with the methods he had already learned from Lavier.

By the time Worsley began teaching in about 1966,[7] his method of treatment, focusing on the Five Element model, was already established. What had happened was that the ancient methods that were abandoned by the Chinese in the 1970s took root and flourished in a most unlikely environment – England.

Worsley's method became known as Classical Five Element Acupuncture and spread to the USA through students who established the Traditional Acupuncture Institute. The lineage tree has since sprouted many branches, with new masters arising to develop differentiations from this original teaching. J.R. Worsley died in 2003 and his work is carried on by Judy Worsley and a wide range of teachers, many of whose works are cited in the text.

Cycles of the Five Elements

It is important to know something of the movement of energy around the Five Element cycle. The fundamental cycle of the Five Elements or phases is known as the *sheng* or generation cycle (see below). It represents a cycle in which each Element gives birth to or generates the next, a cycle which can be illustrated by looking at the seasons in nature.

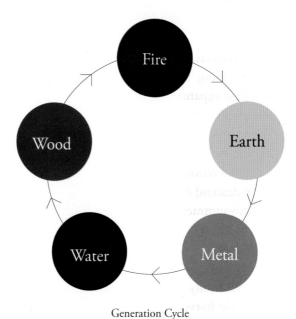

Generation Cycle

Winter is a time of darkness, coldness, stillness and waiting. Nature is preserving its resources, holding its potential for the appropriate time: the seed waiting to sprout. The qualities of Water are quiet, patient waiting, pooling and storing of energy, not rushing to act but waiting for the signal to move. These qualities are what allow the energy of the Wood Element to arise in the spring.

Then, as if a starting gun has gone off, there is sudden, dramatic, dynamic, upward rising and things grow rapidly as temperature and light increase. The seed quickly manifests its genetic blueprint, the map of where the plant is going, what it will become. These are all qualities of the Wood Element.

Wood moves upwards and creates a strong trunk, giving birth to the Fire Element which spreads outwards. This is the energy of summer when everything in nature is bursting outwards to its fullest expansion. Nature is a riot. It is the hottest, brightest, most happening time of year. And the expansion is possible because it has been generated by the Wood.

After the zenith of Fire, the energy of the year begins to descend and generates the Earth Element in the late-summer season. There is a rounding, drooping, sagging feel to nature, a pleasant heaviness. This is the time of harvest when the fruits of the year are made manifest. The extent to which the Fire has fully flourished will determine the bounty of the harvest and the fullness of the Earth.

As the energy of the year continues to fall, Earth gives birth to Metal and the season of autumn. This is the time of year when nature discards what is no longer of use and retains what is of greatest value to life. Trees lose their leaves, plants die after dropping their seeds. There is a garnering of what is most precious. This gathering of deepest value is what generates the return to Water.

If the generation cycle was the only one operating, then the energy would spiral out of control. Therefore, another cycle operates simultaneously. This is the *ke* cycle, or control cycle (see below). Here, each Element exerts a restraining or controlling influence on the next but one in a clockwise direction. This provides checks and balances that ensure dynamic equilibrium among all Elements.

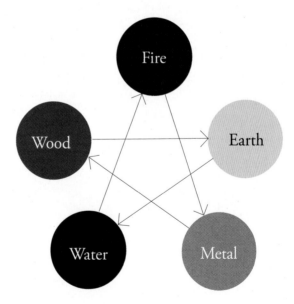

Control Cycle

By looking once again at nature, we can find analogies for this. Water controls Fire the way a bucket of water douses a fire; Fire controls Metal in the way that heat softens and shapes the hardness of metal; Metal controls Wood in the way a knife carves wood; Wood controls Earth in the way tree roots hold soil together; and Earth controls Water in the way banks shape a river's course or create a dam.

When these two cycles are taken together, there is the opportunity for perfect balance and harmony among the Elements. Each Element has a relationship with every other Element. The Five are entirely interwoven and interdependent.

Constitutional Element

The concept of the Constitutional Element is perhaps J.R. Worsley's most significant contribution to the field. Worsley discovered that every person has one Element that has the greatest tendency to go out of balance and that this is also the first Element to go out of balance. Further, he realised that this imbalance causes other Elements to go out of balance in a kind of domino effect. He also concluded that this Element, which seems to be present at or soon after birth, does not change during the course of a person's life. Worsley called this the Causative Factor (CF), namely the Element that is the original cause of imbalance and disease. Some later Five Element practitioners have referred to this as the Constitutional Element, which is the term used in this book.

This Constitutional Element is not always easy to discover. There are many things that obscure it. Symptoms can be a compelling distraction. So too can behaviours and the stage of life the person is in. To find this Element, the practitioner focuses on four main diagnostic tools: the colour in the face, the sound of the voice, the subtle odour of the body and the predominant emotion in the person's life.[8] Each Element has a particular expression of colour, sound, odour and emotion, and ideally these four all appear in the patient. It is enough to have three of these factors to be sure of the diagnosis, but it is seldom easy and sometimes the Constitutional Element is deduced from fewer than three.[9]

When we do find the Element that is the root of all imbalance, then treatment focuses on that Element to bring it back into health and balance. The result of this is that all the other Elements follow it back to balance. During treatment, the other Elements are not ignored, but the treatment keeps coming back to this core Element.

When I refer to treatment, this is usually seen as a patient receiving acupuncture, acupressure or some other Five Element modality. But what I am offering here is a perspective in which all of life can be a source of treatment. You can become practitioner to yourself such that every aspect of your life, including what you eat, what you like to do, your preferences, your emotional reactions, your spiritual beliefs, everything, can become a rich source of inquiry into who you are and why you are the way you are.

In this way, we can come to find our own responses and our own relationship to each of the Elements, to see where we are flowing and where we are struggling. And as we discover the Element of greatest challenge, we find our Constitutional Element. While this Element is indeed a challenge, it is at the same time our greatest potential. It is our life's work. It is why we are here. It is the doorway to unearthing our greatest treasure, the truth of who we are.

Principle of resonance

Imagine a great gong being struck. Its powerful, sonorous note passes out into the universe and all things of a similar vibration pick up the note, vibrating in perfect resonance. Now imagine five great gongs sounding simultaneously, each with its own unique note. Imagine that, according to its nature, every single atom in the universe is resonating to one of these notes. Nothing is left out of this primal harmony.

Similarly, each of the Elements acts like the tone of one of these gongs, vibrating with its own frequency, a frequency that resonates precisely and profoundly in all expressions of that Element: a season of the year, a colour, a sound, an emotion, an odour, an organ of the body, a sense organ, a set of tissues, a psychological state, a spiritual state. They all pick up the note and resonate with its vibration like a great clan singing the same tone in harmony.

Each Element is like the plucked G string of a guitar in a room full of guitars. The vibration of that string causes the G strings of all the other guitars in the room to vibrate, allowing the particular resonance of G to fill the room.[10] If we think of each Element as having a particular vibration, frequency or resonance, then we can understand how all of the associations and correspondences – in fact, everything associated with that Element – will have the same vibration (see the table at the end of this chapter).

When we look inside ourselves, we discover that we are not separate from the grand resonant frequencies of the Universe, and that, just like everything else, we too resonate to all five frequencies. When we are balanced, the five frequencies can find their exact vibration within us, and the result is harmony within and between the Elements.

However, if we are out of balance in a particular Element, there is disharmony not only between the Elements, but within all expressions of the Element, including the particular organs, emotions and aspects of spirit that are associated with that Element. If there is an off note in one correspondence, then all the other correspondences of an Element will also be off note.

The good news is that the corollary is also true. When we address one area of correspondence in our lives, all of the other correspondences will also respond. Thus, we can begin anywhere in our healing and the increasing harmony will flow through to all other areas of the Element. For example, working on the emotion of anger will help to heal the organs of gall bladder and liver, and vice versa. In this example we are bringing the Wood Element into balance, and so all aspects and resonances of Wood will be influenced.

There are many resonances that we could consider, but I have chosen to focus on seven of them.

The seasons of the year are perhaps the most obvious expression of the principle of resonance. Each season has a particular vibration and the way we feel about the season has a lot to do with how its vibration matches our own. Most people have a favourite season and a least favourite season. Some people can't wait for summer to arrive, and feel a sense of loss when it departs, while others hate summer so much they migrate to a cooler climate for those months.

Seasons

On the other hand, there might be all kinds of reasons why people prefer summer to other seasons. Maybe that is when they go on vacation and get away from a boring job for a few weeks. Or it might be because they love summer sports and can't wait for the warm weather to get out there and play. Or perhaps they adore parties and summer is the time when there are lots of barbeques and get-togethers.

If we look at what is common to all of these activities – relaxing on vacation, playing sport in groups, partying with friends – we see that they all have a similar vibration. They are vibrating in resonance with summer and its associated Element of Fire. The way in which you resonate with activities like these gives an indication of the state of the Fire Element within you.

As you move through the year and pay attention to your responses to the changes in the seasons, you will be getting direct information about the state of health and balance of each Element within you. Often, the vibration of the new season will become palpable even before the change in the weather occurs, so it can be very useful to pay particular attention to how you are feeling at the very start of the season.

Senses   The five senses and the sense organs that are their instruments each resonate with an Element. When we focus our awareness on the sense that corresponds to the season, much can be revealed.

The sense of hearing and the ears are resonances of Water. Vision and the eyes vibrate in tune with Wood. Speech (a way we *touch* another's heart) and the tongue are in harmony with Fire. The sense of taste, which we get through the mouth and lips, is in resonance with Earth. Smell and the nose are instruments of Metal.

A heightened awareness of one sensory channel can illuminate our relationship with that sense. This in turn puts us more directly in contact with the Element of that sense. For example, focusing on vision and the eyes puts us in contact with the Wood Element. We can learn things about the way we see and the way we look at and move through the world. These insights can bring healing that flows through to all the other resonances of Wood.

Colour is another expression of the vibration of the Elements: blue or black (Water), green (Wood), red (Fire), yellow (Earth) and white (Metal).

Colours

Take a look at the colours in your wardrobe. What is the most predominant colour? What is missing altogether? Do you tend to wear different colours in different seasons, or in different weather? Do you choose colours to match your mood for the day, or do you choose a colour to change your mood? These choices indicate the influence on us of the different colours and their vibrations.

You can also observe how you respond to the various colours of nature. Do you love the lush green vegetation all around you on a forest walk? Would you rather spend time at the ocean, drinking in its vast blueness? Is your preference for the stark colours of mountains, or the bright red sands of a desert? Perhaps you like many of these colours in nature, but at different times.

As you move through the year, you can pay attention not just to your colour preferences, but also to your response to the colours of nature around you as they change from season to season.

The colour resonance is one of the diagnostic tools of the Five Element practitioner. The practitioner looks for the predominant coloration of the client's face, particularly at the sides of the eyes. Finding this colour is one of the keys to discerning the client's Constitutional Element. The colour is best seen in good natural light, and is often a subtle hue that is seen with 'soft eyes' when the observer is not really trying.

Sounds of voice

The human voice has a tone that reflects an inner vibration. This makes the quality of the voice very useful as a way of finding a person's Constitutional Element. The five voices are described as groaning, shouting, laughing, singing and weeping. Most voices are a subtle combination of these sounds, but everyone has one that predominates.

This predominant sound of voice bears a strong correlation to a person's habitual emotional expression. The way a person speaks has a lot to do with how she is feeling emotionally. Everyone has a predominant emotional pattern and this will be revealed in the voice which becomes a vehicle for the emotion. This is usually quite unconscious and influences the sound of voice whatever the topic of conversation.

Odours

There are five broad categories of odour that correspond to the Elements. These can best be understood by reference to typical smells of the seasons. The odour of Water is putrid, which refers to the kind of smell you might get from a pond. The odour of Wood is rancid, the kind of smell you might get from new-cut grass in spring. The odour of Fire is scorched, like that of parched grass on a hot, dry summer day. The odour of Earth is fragrant, the kind of over-ripe smell that comes from fruit dropped under trees and breaking down in the late-summer sun. And the odour of Metal is rotten, the smell of decaying, composting vegetation in the autumn.

For the Five Element practitioner, odour is a very important diagnostic tool in determining a person's Constitutional Element. Because smell is our most instinctual sense, a person's scent can provide the most direct diagnosis. The odour is not 'body odour', nor the odour of the breath. It is a subtle emanation from the whole body, and can best be sniffed between the shoulder blades, an area that is generally not washed as often as other areas of the body.

The more our health is out of balance, the stronger and more obvious will be our odour. For example, the smell from an unhealthy Wood type will be more like rancid oil than the cut-grass smell of a healthy Wood type. This is because a person's odour arises from the organs that correspond to a person's Constitutional Element not functioning optimally.

The vibration of each Element corresponds to a specific emotion. When we feel a particular

Emotions

emotion, we are like a tuning fork vibrating in resonance with its corresponding Element.

While we all have all of the emotions at one time or another, everyone gravitates to one emotion in particular. It is the emotional groove we tend to fall into much of the time. An assessment of overall emotional temperament provides the fourth and final diagnostic tool used by the Five Element practitioner to determine the client's Constitutional Element. Sometimes these predominant emotions are deeply suppressed and are diagnosed by their conspicuous absence rather than by their presence.

Thus, a person whose most common response to life situations is to become fearful or fearless may be expressing a Water constitution. Someone who is habitually angry or who hides and suppresses his anger might be a Wood constitution. A person who is always upbeat and excitedly joyful, or alternatively flat and depressed could be showing a Fire constitution. Someone who is either overly sympathetic and helpful or selfishly uncaring may be showing an Earth constitution. And a person for whom grief is ever-present or notably absent could be revealing his Metal constitution.

Organs and officials

Each Element has two organs associated with it. Fire has two additional 'functions' which can be seen as subtle organs. Each pair comprises a yin and a yang organ which function together as a partnership. The yang organs are considered 'hollow' because they are like pipes facilitating the passage of a substance.

The yin organs are considered to be 'solid' organs that act as reservoirs of Qi.

When all Five Elements are in harmony, the organs function as they should in harmonious symphony. But when an Element goes out of balance and remains out of balance for some time, this disharmony begins to affect the corresponding organs. These disharmonies tend to take time to reveal themselves in the organs, so by the time a serious health issue arises, the Element has usually been out of balance for quite a while. If we pay attention to the other resonances, we can discover imbalances before the organs themselves show signs of disease.

The *Neijing* is very clear about the harmful effects of emotion on the yin organs.[11] A habitual emotional state goes deep into the body and is injurious to the deeper organs.

Throughout this book you will see frequent reference to the officials of an Element. This is a concept that originated in ancient China and was restored to prominence by Worsley. Each meridian (energy channel) and its corresponding organ also has an official. The twelve officials are personifications of the twelve organs with their functions and responsibilities. The *Neijing* gives them titles and duties as if they were ministers in the imperial court.

When I use the term official, I am referring not simply to the organ or meridian, but to a whole range of functions and areas of responsibility associated with them. These include mental, emotional and spiritual functions as well as physical.

Acupoints

Point names

The variety of meanings suggested by some Chinese characters, together with the large number of synonyms in English, has made for a plethora of translations of the point names. Because this book follows the Five Element tradition, I have, for the most part, chosen to use the translations adopted by Worsley.[12] In some cases I have taken the translations used by Peter Deadman *et al.*[13] in order to echo the text more closely.

Point selection

In narrowing the number of entries to 52 (there are 54 points) I have omitted many important acupoints. My selection has been guided by a wish to include examples of these point categories:

- *Yuan*-source. I have included all source points of the yin meridians, finding these to be powerful, safe and balancing of both excess and deficiency.

- *Luo*-connecting. There are several of these important points which connect the yin and yang meridians of an Element.

- *Shu*. The inner *shu* points which influence the organs and the outer *shu* points which are useful for psycho-emotional conditions, are located on the back along the Bladder meridian.

- *Mu.* These alarm points on the front of the body treat acute conditions and help address emotions.

- Command. Each meridian has five Element points. Here they are used to transfer Qi around the *sheng* and *ke* cycles and are used differently from the five *shu* points of TCM.

- Master points of the Extraordinary Vessels. All eight have been included for their power in balancing these reservoirs of Qi.

- Windows of Heaven. Chosen for their value in working at the level of spirit.

- Meeting points. Points which influence more than one meridian or vessel.

- My own favourites. Some points are chosen for their effectiveness in treating musculoskeletal and myofascial conditions.

When using acupressure on the points, follow the directions for the point and apply pressure for two to three minutes, or until you feel a harmonising of the Qi at the point. I suggest you hold the left side first, then the right.

    I have included a list of points that can be combined with the focal point. All of these are

Treating points with acupressure

points referred to in the book. Related points held in combination are much more powerful than points held by themselves because they act synergistically. Hold the pair for two or three minutes or until you feel them vibrating in harmony together.

Holding the points on yourself is good. Having them treated by someone else is more effective. When you self-treat, you are taking on the roles of practitioner and client at the same time and cannot devote yourself fully to either. Therefore, I suggest you find a partner to work with and take turns to give and receive.

Measurements are often given in *cun*, the basic unit of measurement in Chinese medicine. The cun is a body inch and is a proportional measurement, a division of a longer distance – for example, from the knee crease to the ankle. This means that the cun is slightly different in size from one area of the body to another. However, for our purposes here, the distance across the thumb at the knuckle represents one cun; the distance across the index and middle fingers at the knuckle is 1.5 cun; and the distance across all four fingers at the knuckle is 3 cun.

Table of Resonances

Element	Water	Wood	Fire	Earth	Metal
Season	Winter	Spring	Summer	Late summer	Autumn
Sense	Hearing	Seeing	Speech (Touch)	Taste	Smell
Colour	Blue (Black)	Green	Red	Yellow	White
Sound	Groaning	Shouting	Laughing	Singing	Weeping
Odour	Putrid	Rancid	Scorched	Fragrant	Rotten
Emotion	Fear	Anger	Joy	Sympathy/Worry	Grief
Sense organ	Ears	Eyes	Tongue	Mouth	Nose
Yin organ	Kidneys	Liver	Heart / Heart Protector	Spleen	Lungs
Yang organ	Bladder	Gall Bladder	Small Intestine / Triple Heater	Stomach	Large Intestine
Tissue	Bones	Tendons and ligaments	Blood vessels	Muscles	Skin
Taste	Salty	Sour	Bitter	Sweet	Pungent
Climate	Cold	Wind	Heat	Damp	Dry
Spirit	Zhi	Hun	Shen	Yi	Po

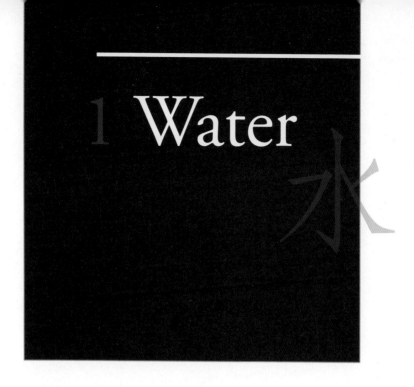

1 Water

The movement of Water is inwards. As the most yin of the Elements, Water will always find the lowest point and come to rest there.

The various ways that water behaves offer insights into the qualities of the Water Element. It is the only natural substance that is found in all three physical states – liquid, solid, and gas – at the temperatures normally found on Earth. Thus, we all have direct experience of the changing nature of water to ice and steam and can observe its indestructibility.

In all its forms, water reveals its power, from the capacity of ice to gouge gorges and sink ships,

The nature of Water

to water's power to erode land and turn turbines, to steam's capacity to drive engines and cause explosions.

In its liquid state, water takes many forms that are very different from one another. Think of the parts of a river, from its beginnings as a spring in the hillside, as a gently babbling brook, as rapids and waterfalls in the mountains, to the broad, powerful, meandering river of the plains and finally to the vast moving depth of the ocean. Think too of puddles, ponds, lakes and wells which show other characteristics of stillness and depth.

In short, water appears in the form of its container, whether it be as a river, lake or ocean; a cup of tea, a bath or a swimming pool; or displaced by a hand, a body or an ocean liner. Water is nothing if not adaptable.

The Chinese character for Water is *shui*. The central stroke represents the main flow of a river while the other four strokes are the whirls, eddies and back currents of the river.[1]

Resonances of Water

Season

Winter

The Water Element is most easily observed in nature as the season of winter. It is the time of year when there is little or no growth, a time of waiting, resting and hibernating. Nature has retreated to its lowest ebb, shrunk to its most minimal, conserving its resources through the long cold night of the year. Temperatures are much lower and in some locations drop below freezing, producing ice and snow.

Winter is the coldest time of the year because at this time the sun's rays hit the Earth at a shallow angle. Also, the long nights and short days prevent the Earth from warming up. Cold and dark are yin qualities and therefore intrinsic to Water.

When does winter begin? This depends on your location and your prevailing climate. In temperate zones, you can expect to feel the beginnings of winter in early November or early May depending on your hemisphere, a month earlier than what is traditionally regarded as the beginning of winter. Yet the first hints of a season tend to have a greater impact upon us. Many people struggle with this transition from autumn to winter which is indicative of an imbalance in the Water Element.

If you live closer to the equator, winter will come later, while if you live closer to the poles, your winter will be earlier. You can look for the signs of winter within yourself: a desire to spend more time indoors where it is warm and cosy, more reluctance to get out of bed when it is dark and cold, reaching into the closet for scarves, gloves, hats and extra layers.

Sense
Hearing

The sense of hearing is closely related to the kidneys which are organs of the Water Element. It is said that if the kidneys are healthy, the ears can hear the five sounds.[2] The tendency of hearing to deteriorate with age is a result of the lifelong decline in Kidney Qi.

Hearing is a sense of rapid response. While it might take a full second to notice something with your eye, turn towards it, recognise and respond to it, the same reaction to sound happens at least ten times as fast. This is because hearing has evolved as our alarm system, operating below consciousness and even during sleep.

Listening is different from hearing. Hearing is simply the act of perceiving sound by the ear. If you are not hearing impaired, this just happens. Listening, however, is something you consciously choose to do. Listening requires attention and concentration in order to derive meaning from hearing. While hearing is a sense, listening is a skill, and both are resonances of Water.

The ears are the sense organs of Water and any conditions that affect the ears such as tinnitus, hearing loss, ear infections and dizziness are indications of an imbalance in the Element.

Colour

Blue
(Black)

Some authorities say blue is the colour of the Water Element, others say it is black, while still others call it blue-black, or even a dark, purplish colour. All agree it is a dark shade.

Water in large quantities, such as rivers, lakes and oceans, is blue because the water reflects the blue of the light spectrum, and also reflects the sky which is often blue. No light penetrates into deep water so there the water appears black.

What is your relationship with the colour blue? How do you feel when you wear it? Do you wear it at particular times? Does it alter your mood? How much do you have in your wardrobe? How much blue is in your home? Too much blue can be depressing for some but it is good to have some of this colour. According to *feng shui* principles, it is beneficial to have something blue on the Water wall of a room, the one in which the entry door is located.

In Five Element diagnosis, blue or black at the sides of the eyes or under the eyes can be indicative of a Water imbalance and may derive from Kidney deficiency. People can get this look when they are very tired, run down or depleted, or if there is some pathology of the kidneys. People of a Water constitution will display this colour even when they are well. Sometimes it looks as if the person is wearing a mask, the dark colour completely surrounding the eyes. It is often dark blue to black, but can appear as a lighter, sky or powder blue.

Sound
Groaning

The sound of voice that represents the Water Element is the groaning voice. This is a sound that is sinking, falling in tone, and which can be indicative of stress or strain. It is a deep note, and one which has little modulation. Of all the sounds of voice, it shows the least variation. It is as if all the inflections have been flattened out. It can sound like water running over gravel. Sometimes it is as if the voice has been drawn out into a longer sound like an old cassette tape that has stretched.

The sound of the groaning voice carries fear, the emotion of Water. Imagine how it is to dread something happening. The groan is the feeling of dread being expressed as a tone: 'Oh no, not that.'

The sound can also reflect an imbalance in the Kidneys which store the *jing* or Essence of life. When there is insufficient energy to power action, a groan of effort is the result. Imagine the sound you might make when getting out of bed after insufficient sleep or anticipating the arrival of a person who is difficult to deal with.

The sound of a person's voice is diagnostic of their Constitutional Element. People who are of a Water constitution will demonstrate this long, low groaning sound in their everyday speaking voice. Like water, it is a sound that finds the lowest level.

Odour

Putrid

The resonance of odour is the third of the diagnostic tools in determining a person's Constitutional Element. Those of a Water constitution have an odour emanating from their skin that is described as putrid. When the person is in good health, this odour is slight and resembles the smell of fresh water. When there is ill health, the odour is stronger and can be like a stagnant pond or even the smell of urine or ammonia.

The odour arises from the organs of the Constitutional Element not doing their job adequately – in this case, the bladder and kidneys not functioning well enough to manage the fluids of the body, resulting in the putrid odour.

The movement of Water is inwards, so it is natural that its emotion is one that sinks and contracts.

Emotion
Fear

Fear is deep, visceral and is experienced low down in the body, affecting the low back, pelvis and legs. In cases of extreme fear, the force of descending energy is irresistible and a person can lose control of bladder and bowels.

Many of the idiomatic expressions for fear are suggestive of its cold, watery nature: a chill down the spine, bowels turning to water, breaking into a cold sweat, blood turned cold, frozen with fear, shaking like a leaf.

All humans experience fear in some way at some time. It is a normal and natural response to danger or threat. It is an instinctual emotion that has helped us survive as a species. However, when fear becomes extreme, goes beyond a reaction appropriate to the circumstances, becomes paralysing or traumatising, or interferes with normal functioning, then this indicates an imbalance in the Water Element.

Imbalance also occurs at the other extreme. When there is a conspicuous absence of fear in circumstances where it would be normal, or when the person repeatedly engages in risky activities without regard for common safety, this is also an imbalance in Water. The legendary daredevil Evel Knievel who holds the record for the most broken bones in a lifetime (more than 433) was a classic example of this type of behaviour.

Emotion is the fourth diagnostic tool in Five Element work. A person of Water constitution will exhibit a relationship to fear that is unusually significant. Fear becomes the predominant emotion of the person's life. The fear will be either very evident or notably absent. Overall, there is something that strikes the observer as not quite right or 'off note' around the emotion of fear.

It must be noted that people who have experienced severe shock or trauma can seem to be Water types. Unresolved traumatic experiences that are held in the bodymind can profoundly affect the Water Element. The emotion of fear can appear to override the emotion of the Constitutional Element. In such cases the other diagnostic tools must be relied upon.

Organs and officials

The organs of Water are bladder (yang) and kidneys (yin), the organs that comprise our waterworks. The kidneys are responsible for controlling the composition and volume of blood by retaining or expelling fluids and minerals, and excreting toxins such as ammonia. The excesses are passed to the bladder which stores the resulting urine until it is expelled from the body. The adrenals are small glands that are located on top of each kidney. While they are a part of the endocrine system, they have an important relationship to the kidneys and the Water Element.

In Chinese medicine, the Kidneys are far more than a filtration plant. They are the storehouses of our *jing* or Essence, both our original Qi inherited from our parents and the Qi we derive from food and breath. The Kidneys also have a direct influence on urination and are seen as the 'gate' which controls this function. Moreover, they control all fluids in the body including the fluids required by other organs such as the intestines, spleen and lungs.

The Kidney official is known as the Controller of Fluids. Kidney is the creator of power, the origin of skill and ability, and the repository of knowledge. This is the yin aspect of wisdom. Its yang counterpart, expressed through the Bladder official, is the clever utilisation of resources stored in the kidneys in a way that will most optimally support progress through life. When these two officials are in balance and harmony with each other, the deep, innate knowing is resourcefully translated into wise living in the world.

Power source point

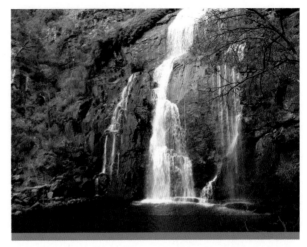

Taixi
SUPREME
STREAM
Kidney 3

We begin our voyage around the points of the Water Element with a potent point of the Kidney meridian. This is the source point of Kidney, *Taixi* – Supreme Stream. The source point of a meridian is often the best point to use because it directly influences the corresponding organ and balances the meridian no matter whether it is excess or deficient. Source points are such safe and effective points to use that they are a good place for beginners to start, and for advanced practitioners to return to.

The source point of the Kidney meridian is located behind the inner ankle. Palpation of this point indicates the condition of the kidneys, while treating it tonifies and balances the functioning of those organs. The Kidneys are the source of yin and yang in the whole body and any deficiency has profound impacts on other organs,[3] so this point provides deep support for overall health.

At a structural level, *Taixi* helps to reduce lumbar pain and stiffness, especially when used in combination with BL 23 in the low back.

The Kidney meridian also influences the urinary and reproductive systems, so *Taixi* can be used to treat frequent urination, cystitis, irregular menstruation, infertility, impotence and premature ejaculation.

The ears are the sense organs of the Kidney, so this point benefits the ears and the sense of hearing. It helps with tinnitus, ear infections and hearing loss. Many of the conditions of old age relate to the decline of Kidney Qi – things such as incontinence, memory loss, hair loss, insomnia and feeling the cold. This point can support a person with any of these conditions and is therefore a boon to the aged.

Supreme Stream steadies the Water Element and can have a very calming effect upon the emotions. It is especially helpful in calming fear, the emotion of Water. This point can settle anxiety, help recovery from highly adrenalised states and aid in healing from frightening and traumatic experiences.

Source points help us to reconnect with our original Qi (*yuan* Qi), that deep reservoir of energy that we were born with and which serves as our fuel tank for life. Since this Qi is stored in the Kidneys, *Taixi* is particularly significant in supporting our connection to this power source. It supports us in realising our potential in the world by aligning us with the positive Water qualities of will, determination, courage, persistence and perseverance.

Holding a point in the season that corresponds to its Element makes it doubly effective. While this Kidney power point can be held at any time, I recommend utilising this resource throughout the winter to support your health at a deep level.

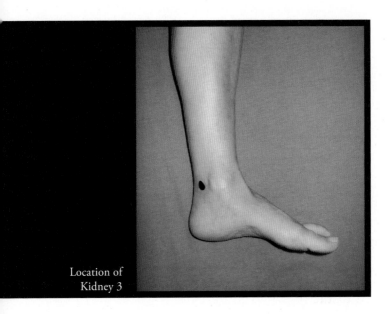

Location of
Kidney 3

The point is immediately posterior to (behind) the inner ankle bone. Find the tip of the ankle and move your finger backwards until you are in the deep hollow between the ankle bone and the Achilles tendon. Feel for a tender spot and use direct pressure.

Combines with BL 23 · BL 52 ·
BL 60 · SP 6 · GV 4

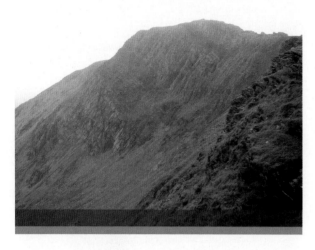

Regeneration mountain

Chinese mythology relates that after the cataclysm of a great flood, the only human survivors were a brother and sister who landed on Kunlun Mountain, rising above the floodwaters. Here they began the repopulation of the world. The two siblings of the story symbolise the primordial yin and yang, while Kunlun represents the central axis of all creation, uniting heaven and earth.[4]

In the human body, this axis of yin and yang is reflected in the fundamental balance between Fire, the great yang, and Water, the great yin. The acupoint *Kunlun* – Kunlun Mountain, the Fire point of the Bladder meridian, provides a means of harmonising the Fire and Water Elements and therefore the yin/yang balance of the body.

When a person feels the cold, there is a contraction of the muscles, but there can also be a tightening of the mind, emotional withdrawal and an evaporation of compassion for others. When the Water freezes in this way and the Fire is doused,

Kunlun
KUNLUN
MOUNTAIN
Bladder 60

* Forbidden during pregnancy

Kunlun is a good point for warming both body and soul.

The distal points of meridians are known for their effects on the whole length of the channel, and this point is particularly strong in its influence upon the whole length of the Bladder meridian. For example, it is well known for relieving chronic back pain, especially in the lumbar region. It combines well with any of the back-*shu* points where pain is located. It is also effective in treating pain in the shoulders, neck and head, especially the occipital region at the back of the head.

Kunlun has a strong descending action, pulling down yang from the upper body – hence its effectiveness for head, neck and back pain. Similarly it treats conditions of the head such as heat in the head, swelling and pain in the eyes, nosebleed and toothache. By causing yang to descend it has a calming and settling influence on the mind. Because of its descending action, it helps to promote labour and is therefore to be avoided during pregnancy.

Another of its functions as a Fire point is in clearing heat from the body. When there is heat in the bladder itself – for example, burning urination or bladder infection – this point is helpful.

Kunlun combines well with K 3 which is its mirror point on the inside of the ankle. This pair brings to mind the flood story in which the brother and sister come together to regenerate the world. Treating the yang of BL 60 with the yin of K 3 is a powerful way to enhance the *jing* or Essence.

When you feel inundated by the waters of life, too exhausted to move, *Kunlun* can raise you to the mountain where a fresh, wider perspective is available and the power of regeneration is possible.

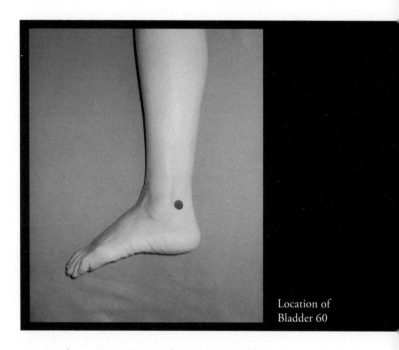

Location of
Bladder 60

The anatomical mountain is the outer ankle bone. The point lies in the hollow midway between the tip of the lateral malleolus (outer ankle bone) and the back of the Achilles tendon.

Combines with K 3 · SI 3 · BL 23 · BL 25

Two extraordinary points

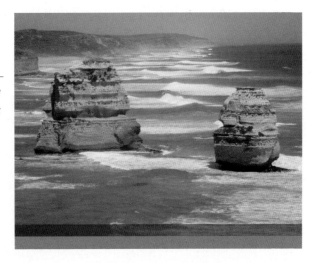

Shenmai
EXTENDING
VESSEL
Bladder 62

Zhaohai
SHINING SEA
Kidney 6

There is no better time to support the Water Element and its meridians of Bladder and Kidney than in the depths of winter. Here we look at two points, one from each of these meridians, two extraordinary points that have wide-ranging effects.

Bladder 62 (*Shenmai* – Extending Vessel) and Kidney 6 (*Zhaohai* – Shining Sea) are like old friends to me, for I have held these points countless thousands of times. I end almost all of my treatments with these points in the feet because they are grounding, very calming and have a balancing effect that ties the treatment together in a complete way.

But I said they are extraordinary points. What makes them so? They are the master points for two of the Eight Extraordinary Vessels, *Yang Qiao Mai* (Yang Motility Vessel) and *Yin Qiao Mai* (Yin Motility Vessel). The Extraordinary Vessels are like reservoirs of Qi. We can think of them as lakes in contrast to the rivers that are the meridians. These lakes do not flow along linear pathways but rather are fields of energy that can be drawn upon or added to by the meridians depending on whether the meridians are excess or deficient.

These Vessels do not have any points of their own, but weave through the points of other meridians like a web. For example, *Yin Qiao Mai* passes through points of Kidney, Bladder and Stomach meridians, while *Yang Qiao Mai* passes through points of Bladder, Gall Bladder, Small Intestine, Triple Heater, Stomach and Large Intestine meridians. When we work with these Vessels, we are influencing all of these associated meridians, bringing balance to them all.

Now, back to our extraordinary points. Each of the Eight Extraordinary Vessels has a master point which exerts a positive, balancing influence upon its related vessel. BL 62 is the master point for *Yang Qiao Mai* and K 6 is the master point for *Yin Qiao Mai*. These points can be held separately or as a pair. I find that holding them as a pair is extremely effective in bringing calm and balance to the whole bodymind system.

In addition, these points have a strong effect upon the Bladder and Kidney meridians and act to balance the Water Element. BL 62 treats chills and fever, wind invasion, headache, neck stiffness, eye and ear problems, bipolar disorder, insomnia and lumbar pain. K 6 treats swelling in the throat, eye problems, insomnia, fright, urinary dysfunction, oedema, irregular menstruation and cold abdomen.

If there are imbalances in the Bladder and Kidney meridians, symptoms are more likely to manifest in the season of winter. But the good news is that by treating these meridians in their own season, the effect is stronger. These two points offer a simple way to bring balance and harmony to your bodymind in the depths of winter.

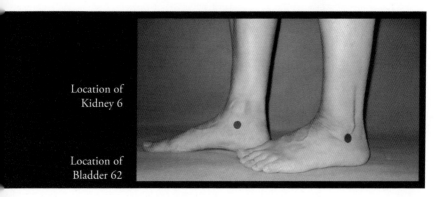

Location of
Kidney 6

Location of
Bladder 62

To locate Kidney 6, find the tip of your inner ankle bone. Measure 1 cun (the width of your thumb) below this to find a slight groove between two ligaments. Use direct pressure.

To locate Bladder 62, find the base of your outer ankle bone. The point is in a slight depression 0.5 cun (half the width of your thumb) below the base of the bone. Use direct pressure.

K 6 combines with
BL 62 · K 3 · LU 7 · GV 4
BL 62 combines with
K 6 · SI 3 · SI 10 · GB 20 · GV 4

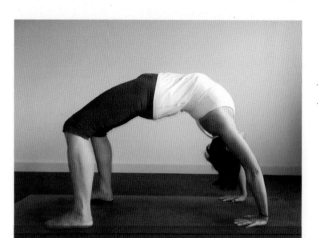

Lumba-go

In winter, cold spreads across the land like spilt water. The colder weather brings challenges for many people, not least of which is the stress it can place on the low back. I tend to see more low back complaints in my treatment room at this time of year. Why is this?

The Kidneys are the storehouses of our Qi. When we push our limits by doing too much, not sleeping enough, not staying warm enough, or even having a lot of sex, we can drain our Kidney Qi. If we do these things in the winter, the strain is all the greater. If there is any imbalance in the Water Element, it is more likely to reveal itself in the winter. One of the ways this can show up is in strain, pain and stiffness in the lumbar region.

There is a point in the low back that is very helpful in supporting the Kidney Qi and the Water Element. It lies on the inner line of the Bladder meridian which runs down the back on either side of the spine. There are points on this meridian

Shenshu
KIDNEY SHU
Bladder 23

called *shu* points which are found at the level of the vertebral junctions. Each *shu* point relates to one of the twelve organs. The word *shu* means transporting, suggesting that the point transports energy directly to the associated organ. At the same time, the condition of the organ is reflected at the *shu* point.

The Kidney *shu* point is *Shenshu* – Bladder 23 – in the lumbar area, on either side of the spine at about the level of the navel. It is the classic point for treating lumbar pain and stiffness, whether acute or chronic. It can be used as a focal point in combination with Bladder points of the leg, particularly BL 40, BL 57 and BL 60, for a powerful treatment for low back pain.

But *Shenshu* is no one-trick pony. It also directly treats the Kidneys themselves and provides access to our deepest reserves of Qi which are stored there. In cases of chronic depletion and exhaustion, it brings about revival by tapping into the person's reserve fuel tank. However, treatment must also be accompanied by changes to the behaviours that caused the depletion in the first place; otherwise, even greater depletion can result.[5]

Shenshu treats all patterns of deficiency of the Kidneys. The Kidneys control fluids in the body, and when they are weak, there can be urinary problems, irregular menstruation or oedema. Yin back-*shu* points such as this nourish their corresponding sense organs, and so BL 23 treats conditions of the ears such as tinnitus and deafness.

Other conditions helped by this point include bone problems, disorders of the uterus, impotence, infertility, weakness or soreness in the knees and feeling the cold, especially in the legs.

A wonderful way to support your low back in the winter is to wear an extra layer of clothing and keep your shirt or top well tucked in. For added warmth, try a *haramaki* or belly warmer which is a tube of stretch fabric that warms the midriff and kidneys.

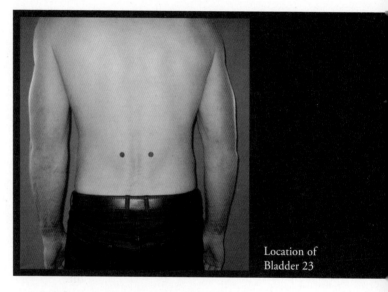

Location of
Bladder 23

The point is in the low back at the level of the junction between vertebrae L2 and L3. This is roughly at the level of the navel. BL 23 lies 1.5 cun (two fingers' width) outside the spine. If you are working on someone else, have them lie face down and apply direct pressure with your thumbs. If you are working on yourself, lie on your back, make fists and place your knuckles into the points. A quick treatment of these points is to sit in a chair and rub your knuckles up and down across these points. It is a stimulating and warming practice on a cold winter's day.

Combines with BL 57 · BL 60 · K 3

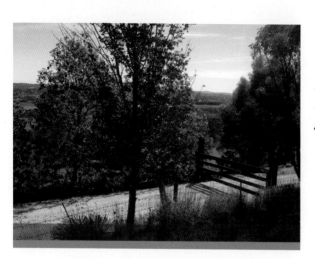

*Fire of the
gate of life*

There is surely no point name more exalted than *Mingmen* – Gate of Life. It goes to the very core of our existence on this plane, our life itself. It is a very powerful point which accesses the gate where we emerge from the void with our Essence, our constitution and our destiny.[6] This point can help us reach our full potential.

Although, according to the Five Elements, the Kidneys belong to Water, they are also the source of Fire in the body, which is called *Mingmen*, the 'Fire of the Gate of Life'.[7] This Fire is needed for our survival as warm-blooded animals and fuels all activity. When the Gate of Life is open, it provides free access to this Fire and there is vitality, sparkle and zest for life. If the gate begins to close, there is diminishment and depletion.

Mingmen is a remarkable point for revitalisation. It can reconnect us with our Essence, raise us to a new level of consciousness, and support the

Mingmen
GATE OF LIFE
Governing Vessel 4

achievement of our highest potential. It is a point that helps to connect us with our original nature.

Lying as it does on the spine between the Kidney *shu* points (BL 23), *Mingmen* powerfully tonifies Kidney Qi and supports the Water Element. If there is timidity, it offers courage; if there is forgetfulness and disorientation, it clears the consciousness; if there is depression or emotional withdrawal, it coaxes the person to re-engage with the world.

Gate of Life addresses the crucial Fire/Water balance in the body, and therefore treats both hot and cold conditions. It clears heat conditions such as a feeling of burning up as well as chills alternating with fever. More commonly, it is used to treat cold conditions such as feeling cold all over the body, especially in the low back and belly, incontinence and abundant, clear urination.

It addresses reproductive disorders such as frigidity, impotence, infertility, irregular menstruation and menstrual pain caused by cold in the uterus. Other conditions include tinnitus, poor memory, haemorrhoids and prolapse of the rectum. It is an excellent point for stiffness, rigidity and pain in the low back and lumbar pain that radiates to the abdomen.

This is an important point of focus in Qi Gong exercises and is known to be one of the three 'tricky gates'[8] on the spine where it is more difficult to move energy, the others being the coccyx and the occiput.

In people who have experienced a chronic, debilitating illness, this point is usually empty and needs considerable attention to persuade it to open. However, it has the power to reconnect with the *jing* or Essence and restore a person to health and vitality, a capacity reflected in its alternate name, Palace of Essence.

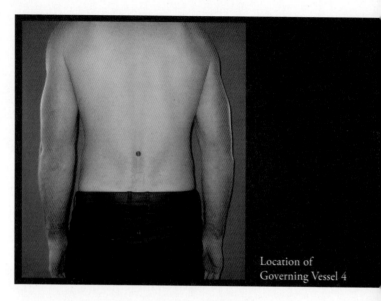

Location of
Governing Vessel 4

On the spine, between the 3rd and 4th lumbar vertebrae, approximately at the level of the navel. Use direct, moderate pressure.

Combines with BL 62 · K 3 · K 6 · SI 3

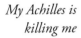

*My Achilles is
killing me*

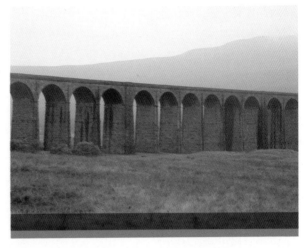

Chengshan
SUPPORT THE
MOUNTAIN
Bladder 57

Tightness in the calf muscles and the Achilles tendon is a condition that affects many people. This includes joggers, cyclists and other athletes who use their legs strenuously. It can also affect people who wear high heels or ill-fitting shoes, those who stand a lot, and those who suddenly take up an aggressive running program after being inactive for a long time. But the condition is not confined to those who are active. People who suffer from Blood deficiency – for example, the elderly and women during menstruation – are prone to tightening of the tendon during the night and so may wake up feeling sore in the calf muscles.

Symptoms of Achilles tendon tightness include cramps, pain and stiffness along the tendon in the morning, pain along the tendon or the back of the heel that worsens with activity, severe pain the day after exercising, thickening of the tendon, bone spur at the heel, and swelling that is present all the time and gets worse throughout the day.

There is a great Bladder point that helps alleviate these symptoms, *Chengshan* – Support the Mountain, which is located in the middle of the back of the lower leg. Sustained pressure here relaxes the Achilles tendon and all the calf muscles that attach to it. This in turn takes pressure off the heel bone where the tendon attaches.

The influence of Support the Mountain extends beyond the leg, for it is an excellent point for pain and stiffness in the lumbar region and for sciatica. When it is held together with Bladder 23, the combination provides an excellent release of the low back. The point also treats haemorrhoids and rectal prolapse.

Did you know that the Achilles tendon is named after the Ancient Greek mythological hero whose mother dipped him in the River Styx to make him invulnerable? Unfortunately for Achilles, the heel by which she held him was not submerged and this remained a vulnerable place. During the Trojan War, Achilles suffered a small wound to his heel and subsequently died. The term 'Achilles heel' is now used to refer to a person's weak spot.

So if calf pain is your Achilles heel, Support the Mountain can come to your aid.

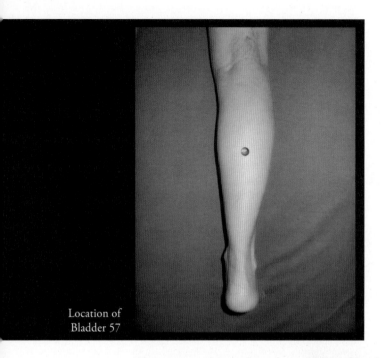

Location of
Bladder 57

The point is located in the middle of back of the lower leg, halfway between the crease at the back of the knee and the ankle. It lies in a depression between the heads of the gastrocnemius muscle. If you press the ball of your foot against resistance, this depression becomes more evident. Use moderate, direct pressure.

Combines with BL 23 · BL25 · BL 60 · GB 30

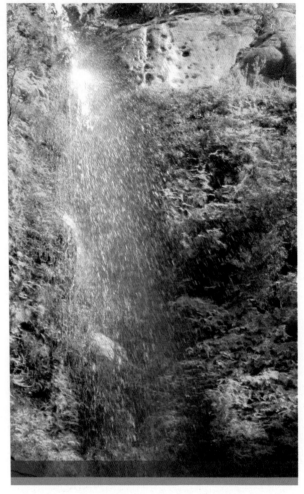

Bubbling spring

In 2009 I began publishing a newsletter about the
Five Elements. The idea for this just bubbled up
one day, like a spring suddenly appearing on a
hillside. When casting about for a title for the
publication, this too just sprang to mind in the
most effortless way. I called it *Bubbling Spring* after
the first point of the Kidney meridian. And like a

Yongquan
BUBBLING SPRING
Kidney 1

perennial spring, this quinterly newsletter pushed its way up, insisting on its publication through four years and 19 issues until it began to morph into a book.[9]

This feeling of something bubbling up irrepressibly from within gave me a direct experience of the nature of the Water Element. Water is the most yin of the Elements but it is not passive. It offers us access to power that comes from true will, wisdom that is borne of stillness, knowing that arises from not knowing.

Yongquan – Bubbling Spring – is the only acupoint on the sole of the foot, the lowest and most yin part of the body which is in continual contact with the yin energy of the earth.

It can therefore be used as a portal through which we can visualise drawing upon the energy of the earth as a tree's roots draw nourishment from the soil. This image of the tree is quite appropriate here since this is the Wood point of the Kidney meridian, one which empowers growth and development to reach our fullest potential.

When a person lacks stamina, strength, will or perseverance, *Yongquan* can help him to draw on reserves in order to get a kick-start. It can restore consciousness and is called for when someone has fainted. On the other hand, it can be used when energy rises aggressively and unrestrainedly, producing conditions such as dizziness, headache at the top of the head, confusion, impaired vision, nosebleed and hypertension.

One of the most important relationships in the body is between the Kidneys and the Heart. The

Kidneys nourish the Heart while the Heart warms the Kidneys. Harmony between the two is one of the main requirements for a peaceful spirit.[10] Therefore, imbalance between Kidneys and Heart is a cause of a range of emotional disorders including anxiety, mania, agitation, restlessness and surges of anger and rage. *Yongquan* treats these conditions by calming the mind and clearing the brain.

It is a very grounding point and can be massaged at bedtime in order to stave off insomnia. Putting your feet in a bowl of warm water for 15 minutes is a wonderful way to bring on sleep.

Yongquan is good for disorders brought on by menopause, including hot flushes, night sweats, anxiety and headache. It also helps Water-related issues such as oedema, infertility and poor memory.

As the Wood point on a Water meridian, this is the sedation point of Kidney and as such moves Qi from Water to Wood around the *sheng* cycle. This is what gives it its power of resurgence. However, the Kidney Qi is rarely, if ever, in excess, and so this point must not be overused lest the reserves of Kidney Qi be depleted.

If you want to put a spring in your step or draw strength from the well of the Water Element, or if you feel exhausted by effort and want to contact your true will, dip your cup in the Bubbling Spring.

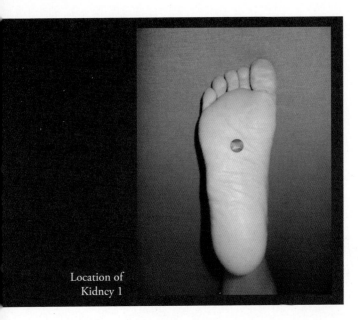

Location of
Kidney 1

On the sole of the foot, the point lies in the depression that appears when the toes are curled. Locate between the second and third metatarsals, about one-third of the distance between the base of the second toe and the heel.

Combines with K 3

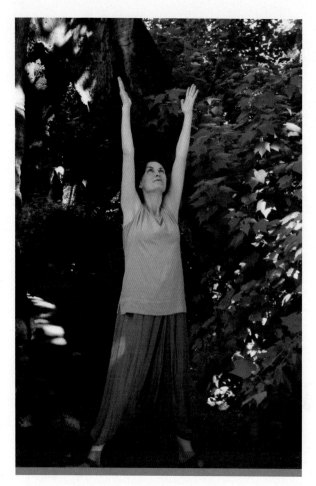

Holding up the heavens

Neck problems are endemic in these days of extensive computer and mobile phone usage, activities which cause us to look down, increasing the force upon the neck. One of the best points for treating the neck lies at the first cervical vertebra, the atlas. In Greek mythology, Atlas was the Titan

Tianzhu
HEAVENLY PILLAR
Bladder 10

who was punished by Zeus for making war on Olympus. He was condemned to stand at the western edge of the world, holding up the heavens on his shoulders. Hence, his name was given to the first cervical vertebra which holds up the head. This Western myth finds a surprising parallel in the point *Tianzhu* – Heavenly Pillar, which lies in the neck on the outer edge of the atlas vertebra and on the lateral border of the trapezius muscle. The cervical spine and the two trapezius muscles can be viewed as the pillars that hold up the head.

Tianzhu is an effective point in treating neck pain, particularly the upper neck. Much upper cervical pain derives from the atlas being misaligned or lacking freedom of movement. This can produce difficulty turning the head, headaches, dizziness or blurred vision, all of which can be treated by this point.

But Heavenly Pillar is far more than a quick fix until you see your chiropractor. The *tian* in the point name means heaven and alerts us to the fact that this is one of the Windows of Heaven, sometimes known as the Windows of the Sky. These points are used to bring harmony between the upper body (heaven) and lower body (earth), and are also used to treat conditions of the orifices (windows) of the head. This window has a particular effect upon the eyes, treating pain and redness of the eyes and chronic tearing. It is also useful for nasal congestion, difficulty smelling, and swelling of the throat with difficulty speaking.

Five Element practitioners also make use of these Windows of Heaven points in ways that address the deeper psycho-emotional aspects of their clients. The positive qualities or gifts of the Element to which a point relates can be called forth from the point and supported in the client. In this case, *Tianzhu* evokes the qualities of Water which include will, courage, endurance, trust and reassurance.

When a person feels unable to hold himself up, feels unsupported to move forward in life or feels that his legs are too weak to support his body, this point is called for. If a person's movement through life is impeded by chronic fear, if he feels frightened by what lies in the future or has grown anxious from an overload of work, *Tianzhu* can bring reassurance that things will be OK. It helps the person to access the true will that arises from *zhi*, the spirit of Water. This can clear the brain, bring a fresh view and an openness to the future. It allows the person to stand tall, hold his head up high and look forward with confidence. At its depth Heavenly Pillar restores trust in the knowledge that true nature is our ultimate support.

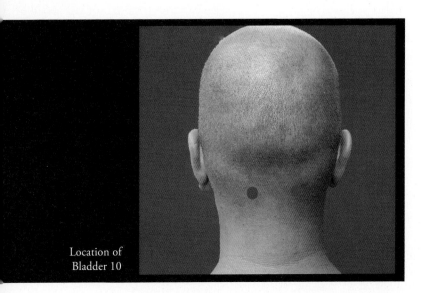

Location of
Bladder 10

At the top of the neck, on the outer border of the trapezius muscle, 0.5 cun below the occipital hollow and 1.3 cun lateral to the midline. Treat both sides at the same time, applying gentle pressure directed slightly towards the spine.

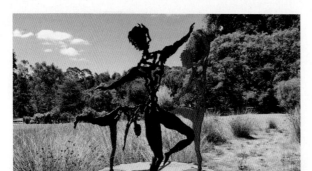

Resurrecting spirit

The character *Lingxu* is made up of two parts, *ling* meaning spirit, and *zu* meaning an old burial ground or a wild wasteland. *Ling* depicts three shamans dancing, supplicating the spirits for rain.[11] The character for doctor or healer also contains the image of a shaman. All of this puts me in mind of Kaptchuk's description of J.R. Worsley, father of the modern Five Element tradition, as the greatest shamanistic healer he had ever seen.[12]

Worsley's own spiritual background predisposed him to regard healing as more than just working with the physical and emotional aspects of a person. His acupuncture work retained the aspects of spirit that were excised by the Chinese Communists when they created what they called traditional Chinese medicine (TCM) in the 1950s and '60s.

Lingxu
SPIRIT BURIAL GROUND
Kidney 24

Most texts of TCM pay little regard to the esoteric aspects of the Kidney points of the upper chest, utilising them simply for physical conditions related to respiration, chest pain and vomiting. In the Five Element tradition, these points can be used to deeply touch a person at the level of spirit. Perhaps the most powerful of these is *Lingxu* – Spirit Burial Ground.

Lingxu, K 24, lies in the middle of a string of points that begins with K 22 Walking on the Verandah and ends with K 27 Store House. These points lie in the region of the heart and are a reminder of the significant relationships between Kidney and Heart, Water and Fire, *jing* and *shen*. K 22 is the exit point of the Kidney channel, where Qi moves to Heart Protector in the *wei-qi* cycle. The remaining points on the meridian represent a mysterious journey of spirit into the darker regions of the human spiritual experience. 'The spirit burial ground can appear as a dark foreboding place to those who have not cultivated the virtues of faith, wisdom and reverence for the will of heaven.'[13]

One of the most profound uses of this point is to treat what is known as a spirit block. This is when the person's spirit had become disconnected in some way from the bodymind. When it appears that a person's spirit has died, when his life appears as a dry and barren landscape, lacking in direction and meaning, when the structures of the ego-self have obscured the true self to such a degree that connection to true nature has been lost, *Lingxu* has the capacity to restore a person's connection to source.

The struggles of the spirit described here recall the notion of the dark night of the soul, first stated in a poem by 16th-century Christian mystic John of the Cross. The main idea of the poem can be seen as the painful experience that people endure as they seek to grow in spiritual maturity and union with God. This journey through darkness to the spiritual light can be seen as an explication of these Kidney points of the chest, and of K 24 in particular.

In treating this point, the intention of the practitioner will determine the level of the client's being that is addressed. If the practitioner uses the point with the intention of clearing a cough and improving breathing, the effects will be restricted to the physical level. There will be a very different effect when the intention is to revive a person's spirit and his connection with the Tao.

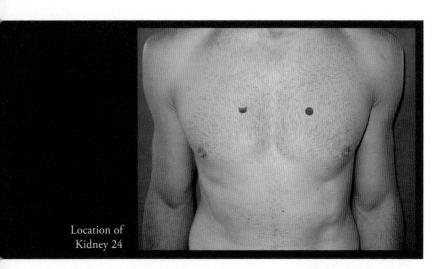

Location of
Kidney 24

Located in the chest at the side of the sternum, the point lies in the third intercostal space and 2 cun lateral to the midline. Note that in males it is one rib space above the level of the nipple. Use direct, moderate pressure.

Combines with K 3 · BL 43

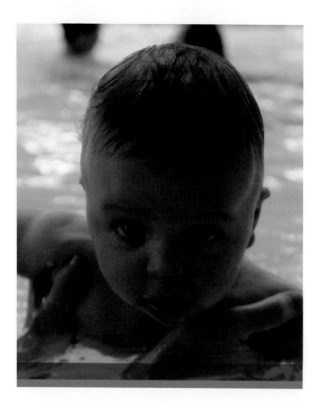

The spirit of Water

Zhi is the spirit of the Water Element. The most usual meaning of *zhi* is will, although it has also been translated as ambition, purpose, determination, knowledge, mind and memory.[14] The will that is referenced here is not that of willpower and effort where there is a forceful pushing and drive to achieve goals. Rather, it works independently of a person's volition, operating virtually below the level of consciousness, a force which moves a person towards his destiny without much conscious thought.[15]

Zhishi
RESIDENCE OF THE WILL
Bladder 52

Kaptchuck describes it as 'the will that can't be willed',[16] meaning that it is the kind of will that allows the person to move forward without pushing the river. A person with strong Kidneys has a strong Kidney spirit, a drive to be alive; one with less Kidney strength may have a lack of drive but overcompensate by pushing himself. Underpinning the *zhi* is the innate power of life itself, life that wants to live, strives to stay alive and survive. It manifests in the human drive to reproduce and thrive, something we have been remarkably successful at as a species.

The classics say that the Kidneys house the *zhi*.[17] Therefore, anything that injures the Kidneys will also injure the *zhi*. Fear that does not flow freely and release from the body will dwell in the Kidneys. Chronic fearfulness, trauma, ongoing stress, penetrating cold, addictions, overwork and insufficient sleep will all contribute to draining the Kidney Qi and therefore the *zhi*. The saying 'burning the candle at both ends' is an apt expression of such depletion.

If the *zhi* is imbalanced, the result is a move to one of two extremes. At one extreme there is a collapse of will, resulting in a lack of drive and determination, listlessness and passivity, weakness, withdrawal and even despair. At the other extreme there is a restless, unrelenting activity that derives from strong ambition and hyper-determination. Put simply, there is either lack of drive or overdrive. Both are symptoms of *zhi* out of balance.

Other possible outcomes of *zhi* imbalance are forgetfulness and memory lapses, the overuse of stimulants to provide false fuel for activity, addictive patterns, insomnia and nervous breakdown.

What does *zhi* look like when it is in perfect balance? Such a person moves forward without seeming to move, as if propelled by some invisible force. This kind of will is unobtrusive and tends to go unnoticed because it is so natural. It is well expressed in the Chinese concept of *wu wei*, the action of non-action. *Wu wei* refers to the cultivation of a state of being in which our actions are quite effortlessly in alignment with the ebb and flow of the elemental cycles of the natural world. 'It is a kind of "going with the flow" that is characterised by great ease and awake-ness, in which, without even trying, we are able to respond perfectly to whatever situations arise.'[18]

Ultimately the highest form of will arises when the personal will is in alignment with the will of heaven. The will of heaven is stored in our Essence (*jing*) and exists within as a blueprint for our highest development. We must align our personal will with this blueprint if we are to manifest our greater destiny. The situations that life presents us with provide the opportunities for understanding the need for this alignment to occur. The more balanced is our *zhi*, the more there will be inner knowing of how this alignment can arise.

There is another important balancing function of the *zhi* which can be seen in its Chinese character, part of which represents the Heart. The relationship between the *zhi* of the Kidney and the *shen* of the Heart is paramount in maintaining the Water/Fire balance which in turn is central to a person's yin/yang balance.

This balanced connection allows the will of the Tao to be mediated by and expressed through the human heart. Harmonious action naturally arises as a willing surrender to the dynamic force of the Tao.

A point that deeply supports the *zhi* is *Zhishi* – Residence of the Will. It is the outer *shu* point of the Kidney and lies on the Bladder meridian. At the physical level, it treats lumbar pain, incontinence, impotence and infertility. More deeply, as its name suggests, it strengthens the will, allowing access to courage, determination and perseverance. It supports a person who is experiencing chronic fear and anxiety which are detrimental to the kidneys and Kidney Qi. In such cases this point can assuage fear by engendering basic trust in the inherent supportiveness of true nature.

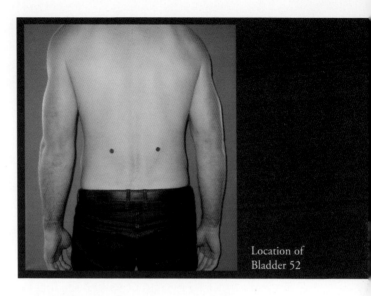

Location of
Bladder 52

The point is in the low back at the level of the junction between vertebrae L2 and L3. This is roughly at the level of the navel. BL 52 is 3 cun (four fingers' width) outside the spine. If you are working on someone else, have them lie face down and apply direct pressure with your thumbs. If you are working on yourself, lie on your back, make fists and place your knuckles into the points.

Combines with K 3 · BL 40 · BL 57 · BL 60

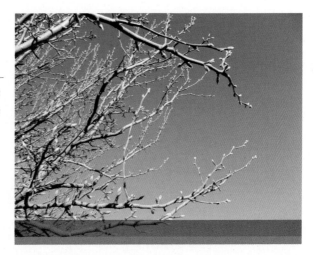

Waking from hibernation

Jingmen
CAPITAL GATE
Gall Bladder 25

Towards the end of winter, the first hints of spring begin to peek though like crocuses in snow. Traditionally, the beginning of spring is March in the northern hemisphere, September in the antipodes, but these changes begin to appear almost a month earlier than this.

According to the ancient Chinese solar calendar, spring starts at the midpoint between the winter solstice and the spring equinox, namely 4th February in the northern hemisphere and 7th August in the southern. The ancients called this 'Establishment of Spring Qi'. From this date, the days begin to lengthen rapidly, temperatures rise and there is an overall quickening in nature.

If you tune in to your own body at this time, you may notice that you too are responding to this speeding up. You may perceive it as a feeling of get-up-and-go, a sudden desire to dust off the hiking boots, clean the mountain bike or get started on spring cleaning. For some it may appear as a restlessness that can only be managed by movement. This is the Wood energy of spring beginning to make itself felt in you.

This is a great time to make plans and start new projects, for the ambient Wood energy will support you in your endeavours. It's a bit like a surfer catching a wave. If you catch the first waves of Wood in February/August, they will add power to your arm as you implement your new plans.

But take care not to rush too quickly to action. Wood energy can be jerky and erratic, and many people suffer tendon and ligament strains in spring as a result of jumping into motion too quickly after a winter of inaction. Make sure you stretch your body before starting physical activity. If you are starting a new project, ensure your plans are sound before you launch into your endeavour.

There is an acupoint which can be very supportive of this transition from Water to Wood. *Jingmen* – Capital Gate – lies on the side/back of the body at the end of the 12th rib. While it is a point on the Gall Bladder meridian (Wood), it is also the *mu* or alarm point of the Kidney (Water). It therefore influences both Elements, helps to smooth the movement of Water to Wood and can ease your passage from winter to spring.

Capital Gate relaxes the sinews and can get you going, stimulating the will to move into action. The point also helps with low back pain, spinal weakness, feeling the cold, lower abdominal cramp or distension, kidney complaints and difficult urination. It is known to support the free flow of Qi in the area after gall bladder removal.

So if it feels like your get-up-and-go got up and went during the winter, support yourself through the transition to spring with Capital Gate.

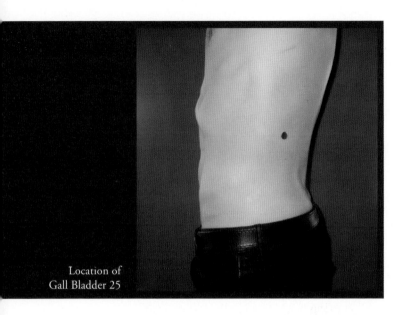

Location of
Gall Bladder 25

GB 25 is located at the free end of the 12th rib. Place your thumbs on your lower back around the level of your waist. Press upwards with your thumbs until you feel the bottom ribs. Follow the ribs down and outwards to the sides of the body until you can feel the ends of the ribs. You are still on the back of your body, but almost to the side. The point is often tender to the touch. Apply moderate, direct pressure.

Combines with K 3 · BL 23

Transition from Water to Wood

As winter draws to a close, there is a transitional period of two to three weeks in which the ambient energy of nature is stirring awake, like a hibernating bear stretching his paws, yawning and thinking of food. There is a sense of buoyancy, as of something rising to the surface of the water.

Even though the temperatures are low, it still gets quite cold at night and the sun still gets up late, something has changed. The days are warmer and some days the warmth is so inviting that you want to find a nice sheltered place and soak up the warmth. Nature is starting to bud and shoot as it responds to this warmth. Overall, there is a sense of things quickening and slowly picking up speed.

But what really characterises this transition is its erratic nature. For a few weeks it feels as if nature cannot quite make her mind up whether it is winter or spring. Stop – Start – Hot – Cold – Yes – No – Maybe. The movement is jerky, like an old train starting its journey where the carriages are jerked a few times before there is a smooth forward movement. In many climates this period is accompanied by gusty winds and driving rain. Some find this weather exciting and exhilarating while others find it disturbing. If you have an extreme reaction towards this transition to spring, then your Wood is probably calling for attention.

When you begin to feel these changes, when you feel the uprising energy within your body as well as observe it in nature, it's time to begin the work of the Wood chapter. Are you ready? On your marks. Get set. Wait for it, wait for it...

Go!

2 Wood

木

The movement of Wood is upwards.

The nature of Wood includes all forms in the plant kingdom, but the quintessential icon of Wood is the tree which sprouts from its seed and rockets upwards in search of light. Its branches splay outwards to fill the space, but the fundamental direction is up.

The many forms that plants and trees take can give us insight into the nature and qualities of Wood. The tiny plant that forces its way up through a crack in the pavement demonstrates Wood's ability to find ways around obstacles to growth. In its early stages, a plant grows rapidly and vigorously, yet also in a jerky series of growth spurts which is another feature of Wood. The weeds that proliferate in the garden show the sheer unstoppable nature of Wood. Bamboo, which bends easily in the wind, is a great illustration of the flexibility of Wood.

Trees can also show us what Wood is like when it is not healthy. Old trees become stiff, brittle and break in the wind. Plants suffering from drought become stunted and gnarled, unable to manifest their full potential. And trees that have died leave their grey bones in a pile, fuel for the next fire.

The Chinese character for Wood is *mu*. The central vertical line represents the trunk of a tree, the horizontal line its branches, the slanting lines its roots.[1] The fact that much of the tree is below the ground is a reminder that a healthy tree and a healthy Wood Element are deeply rooted.

Resonances of Wood

Season

Spring

The Wood Element is most easily observed in nature as the season of spring. Indeed, the very word 'spring' conjures up images of things jumping up suddenly and rapidly, bounding, leaping forth as if from nowhere. Following the quietness, darkness and dormancy of winter, it is as if nature is waking up after a long rest, stretching her arms, feeling her muscles and tendons as she prepares for movement.

We know when the season of spring has arrived because its evidence is everywhere in nature. The grass suddenly takes off and we have to dust off the mower in the shed. The deciduous trees begin to bud and their leaves sprout. We notice the birds beginning to court and nest, and we ourselves begin to feel something rising within in response to this uprising surge in nature, akin to the sap rising in the trees. We start to feel more energy, more interest in getting outdoors, tackling projects and making plans. If we are in tune with the rhythms of nature, this call to movement and action is irresistible.

When does spring begin? This will depend on your latitude and climate zone. In temperate zones, you can expect to feel the beginnings of spring in early February or early August depending on your hemisphere. This is around the cross quarter day of Candlemas in the European tradition, and Groundhog Day in modern American culture. It is the point midway between the winter solstice and the vernal equinox, a time when the lengthening of the days begins to accelerate.

This rapid increase in the daylight hours begins to quicken movement both in nature and in us. Look for the signs within yourself. Pay attention to your predominant focus as it turns from the inward-looking yin qualities of the winter to the outward-looking yang qualities of spring. This shift will be accompanied by an inner sense of something rising upwards in your body. You may feel the bubbling sensation of something coming up the inside of your legs and up the front of your body, filling and expanding your chest with an energy that demands expression.

When you pay close attention to yourself, you will know when spring has sprung. You won't need to look at the calendar or the thermometer; you'll know it from within.

Sense

Seeing

As winter turns to spring, the spotlight begins to move from the sense of hearing to that of seeing. If we have heeded the suggestions of nature and have spent more time looking inwardly during winter, our eyes have been less active. Now, with the longer days, stronger light and much more going on around us, our eyes are called upon to be much more focused

Just as hearing does not automatically imply listening, so looking does not necessarily mean seeing. Our eyes give us the ability to receive visual input. But in order to really see, we must engage in a conscious way with that visual input. This is the difference between dull eyes, and bright eyes.

The eyes are the sense organs of Wood and any conditions that affect the eyes, such as poor vision, eye infections, red or itchy eyes, are indications of an imbalance in the Element.

When we become jaded or bored by life, or we are just going through the motions in a routine way, our looking becomes dulled and we do not really see. The arrival of spring and its Element of Wood gives us the support to see the world with fresh eyes.

Colour
Green

Since the Element of Wood is best represented by the trees and the plant kingdom, it makes sense that green should be its colour. Green is the predominant colour of vegetation. The spectrum of green includes the bright green of new leaves, the emerald green of the fields of Ireland, the dark greens of the northern European forests. It includes the blue-green of the ocean, the bright green of a tree frog, apple green, lime green, pea green and the gemstones emerald and jade.

How much green do you have in your wardrobe? Apparently green is our second favourite colour, so chances are there is quite a bit. If all your clothes are green or you have no green at all, it may be that you need some balance in this. An extreme attitude to the colour green, either an aversion to or an abnormally strong liking, may indicate some imbalance in your Wood.

Do you have green plants in your house? Some green in the home is important for balance. According to *feng shui* principles, it serves to have some green on the Wood wall of a room – the wall to your left as you come into the room.

In Five Element acupuncture diagnosis, the colour green at the sides of the eyes indicates a Wood constitution. Sometimes this green can look a little yellow, making it difficult to distinguish between Earth and Wood constitutions. In this case, other diagnostic indicators become more important to make the distinction.

Sound
Shouting

The energy of Wood is a strong uprising force that demands expression. Of all the sounds that a voice can make, the shout is the most forceful. It gets attention.

When our desires in life are not met in the ways that we would like, we may become frustrated. When we find obstacles in our path that frustrate our forward movement, we may become angry.

The shout is a way that we can discharge some of this frustration. It also lets other people know about our angry feelings. We may even use it to get what we want from others. Sometimes we just need to shout to be heard above the hubbub of everyone else. The shout says, 'Hey, what about me?'

The shouting voice carries the emotion of anger. We all have times when we shout, but when the predominant sound in a person's ordinary speaking voice is a shout, it indicates that they have a Wood constitution. The shouting voice is not necessarily loud. The significant factor is its force and emphasis. It may sound jerky or clipped with an emphasis on final consonants.

Many Wood people actually have a voice that is very quiet, and we may have to strain to hear their words. This is called a lack of shout. It comes about when the uprising and forceful energy of Wood is so suppressed that it begins to disappear from hearing.

The resonance of odour is the third of the diagnostic tools of the Five Element practitioner. This is the subtle odour that emanates from a person's skin. People of a Wood constitution have what is called a rancid odour. When the person is in good health, the odour is not very evident and has a light smell like freshly cut grass. But when the person is out of balance, the rancid odour becomes more evident and can smell like old oil or fat.

Odour
Rancid

The odour derives from the fact that the organs of Wood, the gall bladder and liver, are not functioning optimally in their job of processing oils and fats in the body.

Of all the emotions, anger is probably considered by society to be the most negative. This is because anger that goes out of control can be so destructive. People can get hurt, or even killed. Property can get smashed. Others can become terrified and traumatised.

Emotion
Anger

Because of these potential negative consequences of the acting out of anger, the emotion of anger itself is seen as negative. Yet the emotion itself is no more negative than any other feelings that we may have. In fact, it is the energy of anger that fuels so much activity in the world.

Wood energy is a dynamic, unstoppable force for action. When that force meets an obstacle, the energy builds up and tries to find a way around the obstacle to achieve its goals and desires. Without this force, no action would ever be accomplished. We would just collapse at the first hurdle in our path.

If we relabel anger as an unstoppable force for action, it doesn't seem so negative. We can feel all the frustration and anger we like, as long as we don't turn it into a weapon that harms others. In fact, the more we can stay with the feeling itself, the more it becomes a powerful strength to be ourselves in the world.

Emotion is the last of the four primary diagnostic tools of the Five Element practitioner. When the predominant emotional perspective is from the realm of anger, the person probably has a Wood constitution. For the Wood type, anger is the most difficult emotion to come to terms with. For this person, anger responses to life are extreme. At one end of the scale, there may be a response of fury and rage at the least provocation. At the other end of the scale, the person is unable to be angry even when it is appropriate – for example, when they are being unjustly treated. It is difficult for the Wood type to be in a place of balance around anger.

Organs and officials

The organs of Wood are gall bladder (yang) and liver (yin). The liver has more than 500 functions, the most important of which are the metabolism of protein, carbohydrate and fats, the production of bile to aid digestion, and the detoxification and purification of blood. The gall bladder serves as a temporary store for bile secreted by the liver. Its release is triggered by the ingestion of a meal containing fats.

In Chinese medicine the Liver has the functions of storing Blood, ensuring the smooth flow of Qi and Blood throughout the body, controlling the sinews and housing the *hun* or ethereal soul. It manifests in the nails, opens into the eyes, controls tears, and is affected by anger.[2] Meanwhile, the Gall Bladder is responsible for nourishing the tendons and ligaments, especially in the limbs, allowing for smooth movement in the world. It is also responsible for decision making. 'The Gall Bladder is like an impartial judge from whom decisiveness emanates.'[3]

The Liver official is responsible for making plans and seeing the big picture. It is often personified as an army General who surveys the whole scene, sees the best way forward and strategises a grand plan to achieve his goals. His partner, the Gall Bladder official, is like the Chief of Staff who is responsible for making decisions on the ground and taking the day-to-day actions that will carry out the General's plan. Together, the Wood officials take the potential inherent in Water and utilise it to implement action in the world.

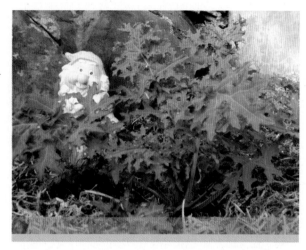

Is life worth living? It all depends on the liver

Taichong
SUPREME
RUSHING

Liver 3

This witty word play by 19th-century American philosopher William James serves as a reminder that the health of the liver organ is of utmost importance in living a healthy life. If you want to live, you have to have a liver.

Of the many functions of the liver, the most important include synthesis of amino acids and cholesterol; metabolism of carbohydrates, proteins and fats; and the production of bile which assists digestion in the small intestine. The liver plays several roles in the regulation of the blood, breaks down insulin, breaks down toxic substances and allows them to be excreted. In short, the liver supports almost every other organ in the body.

In Chinese medicine, the Liver is the yin organ of the Wood Element. Since spring is the season of the year in which Wood energy is at its peak, spring is the best time to support this organ. Eat plenty of fresh dark green vegetables. Kale, like that pictured in my garden in spring, is one of the best foods to cleanse the liver. Sour foods such as lemons and limes, and fermented foods such as sauerkraut are also terrific. If you've been thinking of doing a liver cleanse, then start right now.

Perhaps the best acupoint to aid your dietary efforts is *Taichong* – Supreme Rushing. This is one of the great tonic points of the body. As the source point of the Liver meridian, it directly treats the organ itself. It also influences many conditions associated with the Liver and the Wood Element. For example, it treats conditions of the eyes which are the sense organs of Wood. It helps with abdominal distension and pain, menstrual irregularities, urinary and genital conditions, all of which occur in areas of the body through which the Liver meridian passes.

Supreme Rushing helps ease insomnia and disrupted sleep as well as headaches that are the result of Liver Qi stagnation. If you've eaten too much fatty food, drunk too much alcohol or taken a lot of medications, this point will support their metabolism by the Liver.

At the psycho-emotional level, anger is the emotion of the Wood Element. Anger that does not flow freely tends to lodge in the Liver. Therefore, this point can soothe agitation, irritation, frustration and anger. It calms the mind and imparts courage and clarity. Where there is depression caused by suppressed anger and frustration, it can liberate a person's aliveness and fuel the upward-rising energy necessary to allow active engagement with the world.

If you want to give your Liver a jump start this spring, Supreme Rushing can rush to your aid.

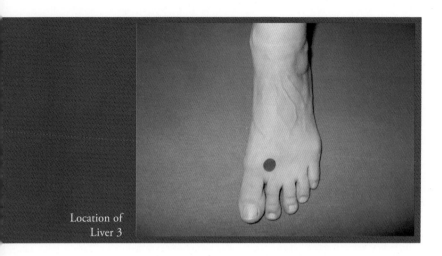

Location of
Liver 3

The Liver source point lies on the top of the foot in a large hollow between the first and second toes, halfway along metatarsal bones. There will probably be a sensitive spot. If the liver is very congested, the point itself may feel thick and swollen. Use moderate, direct pressure.

Combines with LV 14 · GB 34 · BL 47

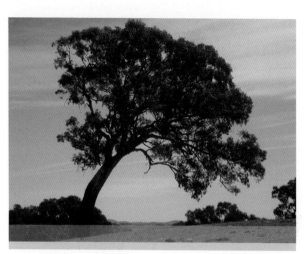

How flexible are you?

The sinews of the body, the tendons and ligaments, are the province of the Wood Element, and particularly of the Gall Bladder. When Wood is healthy, there is strength and flexibility in these tissues, joints move freely and the body moves smoothly in space. When Wood is wobbly, there can be stiffness in the joints and tightness in the tendons which make movement slow and painful. Sometimes the problem is the opposite: the tendons and ligaments are too loose, the joints lose their structural integrity and bones do not hold their alignment.

Yanglingquan
YANG MOUND SPRING
Gall Bladder 34

The concept of flexibility extends beyond the physical structures to the psychological level. Inflexible attitudes and beliefs can also point to an imbalance in Wood. Healthy trees bend and sway with the wind; as humans, we need to be able to adapt flexibly to changing conditions if we are to move smoothly through life. On the other hand, some people are so over-flexible and accommodating towards others that they lose sight of themselves. If you bend over backwards for people, you are likely to hurt your back!

Yanglingquan – Yang Mound Spring – is considered to be the master point for treating the tendons and ligaments and bringing smooth flexibility to them. The point nourishes the tendons, relieves spasms and cramps, especially along the pathway of Gall Bladder – head, neck, shoulders, sides of the ribcage, hips, and sides of the legs. It also treats sciatica which refers down the side of the leg.

There is a saying in Chinese, 'He has a small gall bladder', which refers to a person who is timid, shy, indecisive, anxious and wary. Yang Mound Spring is a wonderful point for strengthening the mind and spirit in this arena, supporting the person to be bold, confident and decisive in the world.

Gall Bladder 34 also supports its partner organ of Liver, treating nausea, vomiting, indigestion, jaundice and hepatitis. At the emotional level, it can move stagnant emotions which lodge in the Liver, such as depression, frustration, irritability, anger and confusion.

If you want to maintain a flexible body and an adaptable mind, treat yourself to a little Yang Mound Spring.

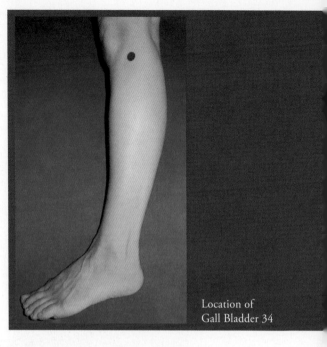

Location of
Gall Bladder 34

The point lies below the outside of the knee in a depression inferior (below) and anterior (in front) to the head of the fibula. Slide your finger up the side of your lower leg until you find a bony prominence below the knee. Move one cun diagonally forward and down until you feel a tender spot in the depression where the fibula meets the tibia. Apply firm, direct pressure.

Combines with GB 21 · GB 41 · LV 3

Keep your shoulder well

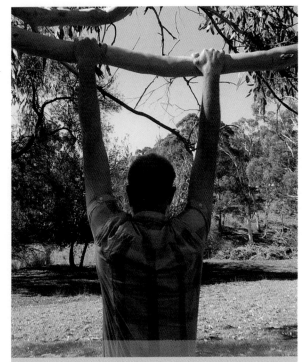

Jianjing
SHOULDER
WELL
Gall Bladder 21

* Caution during pregnancy

I had my first experience of acupressure 30 years ago when I attended a talk. As part of his demonstration, the teacher pressed his thumbs into the tops of my shoulders, causing a release of energy that bolted through my whole body. It really got my attention. I later discovered that he was working a point on the Gall Bladder meridian, *Jianjing* – Shoulder Well. The reason that it was such a powerful point for me was that I had spent the previous seven years teaching in high schools and had accumulated more than a little tension in my shoulders. Layers of frustration and anger had been tightly controlled by fear of prosecution if I should let it out on my students.

Many of the stresses of modern living find their way into the shoulders. The responsibilities of life can seem to weigh on the shoulders like the straps of a heavy backpack. Most people have some tension in these points which is why a shoulder massage usually feels so good.

Tightness in the shoulders affects the smooth flow of Qi along the Gall Bladder meridian. It limits the range of neck movement and so constrains clear vision and perspective. Likewise, it inhibits the free movement of the arms which are the means of taking action in the world.

The official of Gall Bladder is sometimes referred to as the Chief of Staff. While the Liver official, the General, is responsible for planning and strategy, the Gall Bladder official carries out the plans, riding hither and yon to oversee their implementation. If we live a busy life, we are constantly multitasking and keeping all the balls in the air. When we live a life of *doing* and lose touch with *being*, congestion in the Gall Bladder channel can result. The tops of the shoulders have a particular tendency to become congested.

Jianjing is a meeting point with the Stomach and Triple Heater meridians and the Yang Linking Vessel, making for a deep concentration of meridian Qi at this point. It has a strong descending action, drawing congested energy down the body. For this reason it is not recommended during pregnancy, although it is useful to assist labour and promote lactation. It is also supportive after a miscarriage.

When there is ongoing frustration, anger, resentment and rigidity, these emotions can become stuck in the neck and shoulders. The whole neck can become rigid from these bottled-up feelings. Shoulder Well can relieve such a bottleneck of energy, especially when combined with GB 20 at the top of the neck. It eases neck stiffness, treats shoulder and upper back pain, and helps to lower blood pressure.

When the tension in your life is creating boulders on your shoulders, take your bucket to the Shoulder Well.

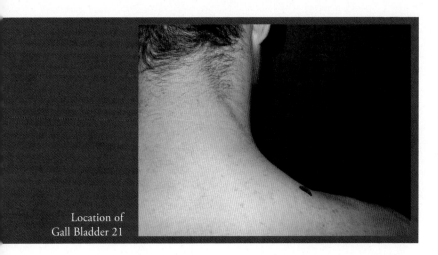

Location of
Gall Bladder 21

The point is on the crest of the shoulder, midway between the base of the neck and the tip of the shoulder (acromion). Reach up and press your middle finger into the tightest part of the trapezius muscle on your opposite shoulder. It is difficult to apply deep pressure yourself, so get a friend to press his thumbs into the points while you are sitting or lying down. Apply firm, downward pressure. In cases of extreme tightness, you can rub or knead the muscle first before applying static pressure. For self-help, there are cane-shaped tools available which allow you to apply leveraged pressure.

Combines with GB 20 · GB 34 · GB 41 · ST 36

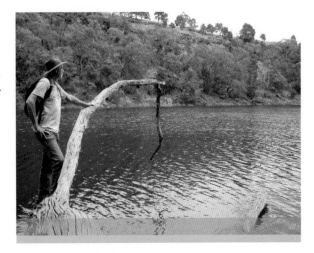

Neck release

Fengchi
WIND POND
Gall Bladder 20

I spend more time holding this point on my clients than any other and I use it in most sessions. This is partly because in my early training I learned a neck release that concluded with this point. In doing thousands of neck releases over the years, I have come to see how helpful it is for most people to have the upper cervical region released. Most people relax and some even fall asleep with this point. It is a great boon in our modern, stress-filled world.

What makes this such a significant point is that it is not only a Gall Bladder point, but also a meeting point with the Triple Heater meridian, Yang Motility Vessel and Yang Linking Vessel. By affecting two meridians and two vessels at the same time, this point has wide-ranging effects.

Its name, *Fengchi* – Wind Pond, tells us two things. First, it is like a pond or pool, lying as it does in the little hollow between the trapezius and sternocleidomastoid attachments at the occipital bone. Treating this point releases tension in these two important muscles of the neck, taking pressure off the cervical spine.

Second, we learn that it is a pond that accumulates wind, the climatic condition of the Wood Element. Wind can penetrate the body from the outside as a pathogenic factor, collecting here before invading the body more deeply. This includes strong winds in nature but also draughts, especially from air conditioning. The most common symptoms of wind invasion are stiff neck and headache, but it can also cause sneezing, runny nose, scratchy throat, fever, aching joints and facial paralysis. *Fengchi* treats these symptoms by driving out the wind from the place where it entered.

Wind can also develop internally as a result of disharmony in the Liver, producing symptoms such as tremors, tics, convulsions, severe dizziness and numbness. *Fengchi* also treats these conditions.

More generally, it is perhaps the best point for clearing the head because of its effect on the sensory orifices, especially the eyes. It treats vision and eye disorders, dizziness, vertigo, deafness, tinnitus and sinusitis. It relieves pain in the head, neck and shoulders, particularly occipital headache.

The head is said to be the residence of the yang.[4] Because GB 20 is a point of the Yang Linking Vessel which unites all six yang meridians and the Governing Vessel, it has a profound influence on rising yang. It causes any pathological Qi to descend and is therefore the pre-eminent point for headaches of all kinds and dizziness of any origin.

It has a powerful effect on the brain, bringing clarity to the eye and mind and enabling a clearer view of the world. It clears confusion, strengthens concentration, aids memory and supports the making of good judgements and decisions. If you can't see the wood for the trees, Wind Pond will help to broaden your perspective.

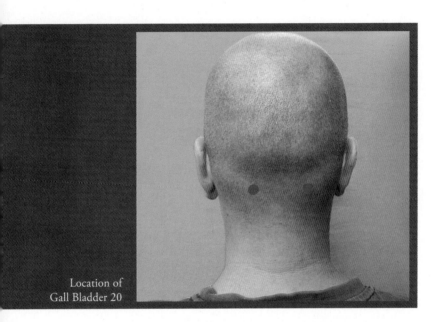

Location of
Gall Bladder 20

Below the occiput (the ridge at the back of the skull) and midway between the midline and the mastoid process. The point lies in the hollow formed by the origins of the trapezius and sternocleidomastoid muscles, approximately 1.5 cun lateral the occipital hollow (GV 16). Apply direct pressure or angle towards the opposite eye. An effective method is to cradle the person's head in your hands and apply pressure with the middle fingers to both points simultaneously. This has the effect of applying a gentle stretch to the neck which has a relaxing effect upon the whole spine.

Combines with GB 21 · GB 41

Gate of hope

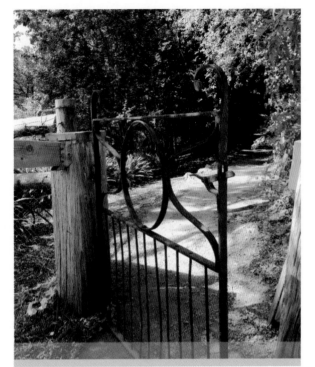

Qimen
GATE OF HOPE
Liver 14

Depression is an all too common condition these days. Feelings of flatness, hopelessness, pointlessness or simply a feeling of being down and blue are some of the characteristics of depression. From the perspective of Chinese medicine, one of the causes of depression is an imbalance in the Wood Element arising from stagnation in the Liver Qi, which can in turn be a result of suppressed anger. Since anger is the emotion that corresponds to the Wood Element, constricted anger can affect its yin organ, the Liver, resulting in a suppression not only of anger, but of vibrancy, aliveness, motivation and the willingness to move boldly through life.

When it is healthy, Liver Qi rises up from the feet and legs, through the groin and abdomen to the chest, empowering action and engagement with life. It is akin to the sap rising up a tree to nourish its branches and leaves. A common place for this uprising Qi to become stuck is in the chest at the exit point of the Liver meridian, *Qimen* – Gate of Hope.[5]

When this point becomes blocked, there can be constriction in the diaphragm leading to frequent sighing. There may be pain, distension and fullness in the chest as well as epigastric pain, nausea, reflux and vomiting.

At the psycho-emotional level, blocked Qi at *Qimen* may result in an inability to see the way forward in life, feelings of gloominess, hopelessness and resignation. Opening the Gate of Hope can expand the horizons, allowing a person to see the limitless possibility that life has to offer. It invigorates the Liver official whose task is to roll out plans based on the big picture. It provides support to meet the challenges of the world with zest and vigour, direction and purpose.

When Qi moves freely from here to the next point in the cycle, Lung 1, there is inspiration to aspire to greater things, support for the planning and creativity to express these aspirations in the world, and the strength and flexibility to carry them forward. All of these qualities are the gifts that are available to us when our Wood Element is in balance.

At the level of spirit, the spiritual issue of the Wood Element is finding one's true path in life.

What is the essential orientation and direction of
your particular existence? What is the path through
life that best expresses and unfolds your individual
soul? Gate of Hope can support you as you ponder
these existential questions.

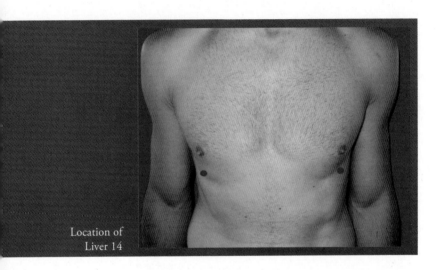

Location of
Liver 14

The point is located in the sixth intercostal space,
on the nipple line – 4 cun lateral to the midline.
First locate the tip of the xiphoid process which is
the knob of cartilage that attaches below the breast
bone. Move your finger across the ribcage until you
are in line with the nipple. Then come up until you
land in a rib space. On a woman, this is the rib
space below the breast. The point will probably be
sensitive. Use moderate, direct pressure.

Combines with LV 3 · BL 47 · LU 1

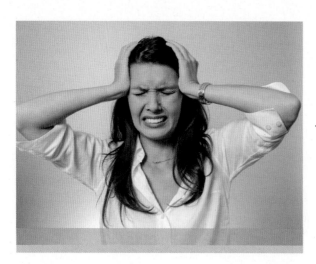

Tears of frustration

Most of us have had the experience of becoming so frustrated with something or someone that we burst into tears. Anger and frustration become so pent up that they find a release through crying. Such an emotional state is usually an indication of an imbalance in Wood which can be treated by the Gall Bladder point *Zulinqi* – Foot Above Tears.

Zulinqi
FOOT ABOVE TEARS
Gall Bladder 41

Wood that is healthy and moving freely aids us in finding a clear path around the apparent obstacles that life presents, like the plant that pushes its way through the cracks in the footpath. When Wood is not healthy, there are two polarised responses to obstacles: a repeated pushing against an immovable impediment resulting in frustration; or a collapse into inaction, defeat and giving up.

Zulinqi helps to resolve such polarised attitudes by strengthening all the resonances of Wood. It supports new ventures and putting your best foot forward as you move into action; provides a clear perspective of where you are and where you are headed; and helps with making good judgements and taking bold decisions. It treats Gall Bladder timidity where a person is fearful of taking action, and relieves depression caused by collapsed Wood. It helps to settle the person who is continually angry, frustrated and resentful.

Zulinqi supports the Wood in two ways. First, it smooths and clears the Gall Bladder channel, the complex pathway that begins at the outer corner of the eye and traverses the head, neck, shoulders, ribcage, hip, side of the leg and foot. Clearing this channel supports flexibility of the mind and body in negotiating a smooth path through life. Second, the point strongly supports the smooth spreading of Liver Qi, allowing it to ascend to fuel action and promote free respiration.

As the exit point of Gall Bladder meridian, it drains congested Qi from the upper reaches of the channel, especially from the head. Holding this point is like taking the plug out of a bath to drain it. Thus, it can treat headaches, especially at the back and top of the head, visual distortion, dizziness and tinnitus.

As the Wood point of a Wood meridian, Foot Above Tears has an energising effect on the Element. It shakes the tree, rouses the Wood: Wake up, let's go, it's time to move! Element of the Element points such as this also function as horary points (from the Latin *hora* meaning hour). According to the Chinese meridian clock, the high tide of the Qi flow passes through Gall Bladder meridian between 11pm and 1am. Therefore, the point has a greater influence during this time. People who have difficulty falling asleep at this time of night may find the point conducive.

Zulinqi has another role as the master point of the *Dai Mai* (Girdling Vessel), one of the Eight Extraordinary Vessels, and the only one that does not have a longitudinal trajectory. It passes round the back at the waist, dropping lower towards the pelvis in front, like the low-slung belts that were iconic fashion items in the '80s. This vessel binds the Penetrating and Conception Vessels, and the Liver, Spleen and Kidney meridians, all of which influence the menstrual cycle. This powerful master point therefore regulates menstruation and treats PMT, which so often comes with tears. It also helps with infertility, vaginal discharge, abdominal fullness and lumbar pain. It relieves the low back and hip pain of pregnancy.

Locally, it treats pain and swelling on the top of the foot, and helps to heal the most common of foot fractures at the fifth metatarsal.

Some say that frustration is a motivating force that leads to success. I would suggest it is a sign that Wood is getting stuck. *Zulinqi* can help to unblock the logjam and free the energy for directed, purposeful action.

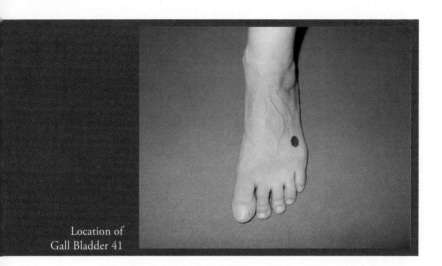

Location of
Gall Bladder 41

On the top of the foot, in the depression below the junction of the 4th and 5th metatarsals. Draw up between the fourth and fifth toes, cross over the tendon of extensor digitorum longus and drop into the hollow. Apply direct pressure. The point is often quite sensitive.

Combines with GB 21 · GB 34 · LV 3 · TH 5

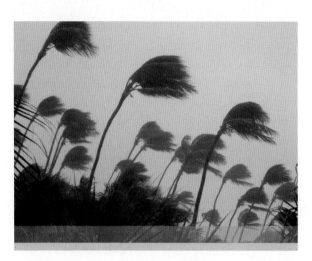

*Surviving the
spring wind
invasion*

Strong, gusty winds are a hallmark of spring in many places. Where I live in the Adelaide Hills, last spring saw blustery winds toppling trees all over the region and I lost my broad bean crop when the slender canes snapped in the gale.

Fengdu
WIND PALACE
Governing Vessel 16

Wind can have a detrimental effect on humans as well as vegetation. In Chinese medicine there are conditions known as wind invasion and wind stroke where wind penetrates the body. All of us are familiar with heat and cold invading the body, producing heatstroke and chills, but it is less well known that wind, the climate of the Wood Element, can also enter the body and produce symptoms of imbalance.

Some people love the wind and are impervious to its influence while others are sensitive and dislike going out in windy weather. Some are so sensitive that even looking out of the window at wild, windy weather can bring up feelings of unease.

One of the classic places for wind to invade the body is through the neck, particularly in the upper part where the skull joins the cervical spine. Here lies the acupoint *Fengdu* – Wind Palace, a point on the *Du Mai* (Governing Vessel) that is particularly susceptible to wind invasion.

Symptoms of pathogenic wind invasion include pain and stiffness in the neck, headaches, mental disturbance or fogginess, dizziness, blurred vision, shivering, sweating, aversion to cold and a general feeling of heaviness in the body. This condition can arise from prolonged exposure to blustery winds. It can also be caused by sitting or lying in a draft or in air conditioning.

Fortunately, the wind can be encouraged to exit at the same place it entered. Sustained pressure at Wind Palace allows the wind to clear from the body. You can use finger pressure, but another useful technique is to lie on your back with a tennis ball pressing into the occipital hollow. The weight of your head creates the pressure and you can relax without having to do anything.

If you are prone to neck problems, I recommend wearing a scarf when going out into the wind. Make sure it covers the very top of your neck where the wind likes to sneak in. If you have a very strong dislike of the wind, it may be that there is some internal wind that needs to be cleared. Work on Wind Palace for a few minutes each day over the next week and see if you become less disturbed by the wind.

Another significant function of *Fengdu* is as one of the Windows of Heaven. Windows points are effective in treating conditions of the head, neck and the sense organs. At a deeper level, *Fengdu* nourishes the brain and can help to widen a person's horizon and keep them focused on the path ahead. When there is depression, it can revitalise the connection with spirit and encourage outward vision and moving on with life.

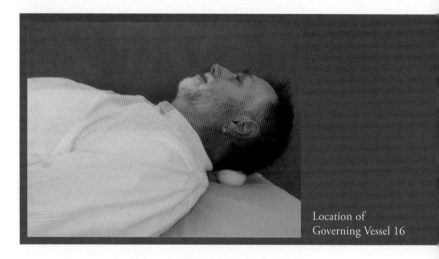

Location of
Governing Vessel 16

The point is located on the midline at the top of the neck in the large hollow immediately below the external occipital protuberance. Use your middle finger to trace up the middle of the back of your neck until you encounter the large bump at the back of the head. The point is in the depression immediately below. You can hold it with upward-directed finger pressure, lie on a tennis ball or ask someone to hold the point for you while you lie back and relax.

Combines with GB 20 · SI 3

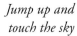

*Jump up and
touch the sky*

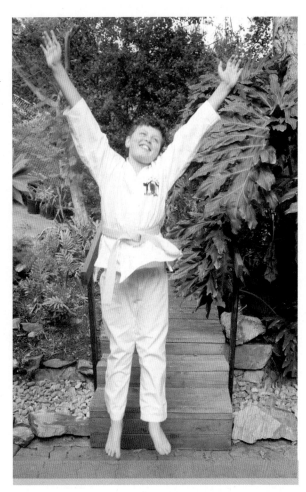

Huantiao
JUMPING CIRCLE
Gall Bladder 30

I love the name of this point. *Huantiao* – Jumping Circle – conjures images of ultra-flexible dancers leaping nimbly, twisting spectacularly in mid-air and landing with grace. It suggests strength, stamina, flexibility and a vigorous engagement with life. It is the very model of healthy Wood.

As a bodyworker, I find this point indispensable in treating hip pain and stiffness, and especially sciatica. It influences not only the hip but also the whole of the leg. For example, it treats knee stiffness where flexion and extension of the knee are limited. It addresses thigh pain and numbness in the leg, and promotes circulation of blood throughout the lower limb. Furthermore, it treats pain in the lumbar region as well as the sides of the ribs, which lie along the pathway of Gall Bladder meridian.

It is the go-to point for sciatica, a condition that produces pain through the buttock and down the back of the leg. Sciatica is caused most commonly by a herniated (bulging) disc pressing on the sciatic nerve as it emanates from the spine. Nerve entrapment can also be caused by spinal bone spurs and displaced lumbar vertebrae. Sciatica can also result from a tight piriformis muscle pressing on the nerve as it passes through the buttock. *Huantiao* treats sciatica arising for any of these situations.

Ma Danyang, the 12th-century Taoist luminary, included this point in his now famous Eleven Points Shining Bright as the Starry Sky, indicating its use for 'pain in the leg from hip to calf and repeated sighing in grief when turning'.[6] Today practitioners regard it as unrivalled in importance for the treatment of disorders of the hip joint and buttock, whether from traumatic injury or stagnation of Qi.[7] It strengthens all of the tendons and ligaments, the tissues of the Wood Element.

Huantiao is also a meeting point with the Bladder meridian, meaning that its effects can be felt along the pathway of Bladder channel as well as Gall Bladder. Thus, it can treat pain in the low back through which the Bladder meridian passes.

Besides these structural effects on the body, *Huantiao* also eliminates wind, cold and damp heat, making it effective in treating skin rashes in the lower body, itchy anus and groin, urethritis and vaginal discharge. In a systemic way, it tonifies Qi.

Wood likes to move. When our Wood is balanced, the sinews of the body are supple, bestowing ease of movement. Our legs take us where we will. We are free to roam through life as the clouds wander the skies. *Huantiao* grants us this range of motion.

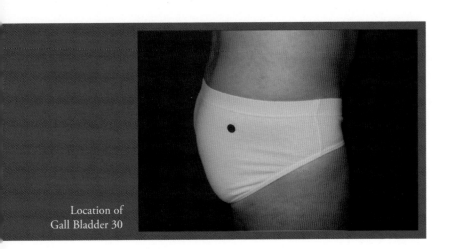

Location of Gall Bladder 30

When a person squats down in preparation for a jump, a semi-circular depression appears at this point.[8] This hollow is located two-thirds of the distance from the sacral hiatus (bottom of the sacrum) to the tip of the greater trochanter of the femur (hip bone). It is found most easily with the person lying on their side with the leg bent. Apply firm, direct pressure.

Combines with GB 34 · GB 41 · BL 57 · BL 60

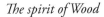

The spirit of Wood

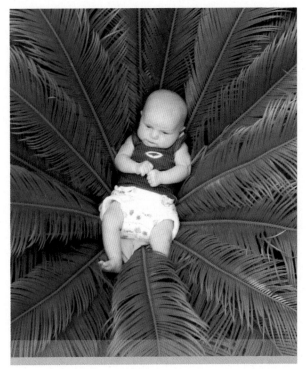

Hunmen
GATE OF THE
ETHEREAL
SOUL
Bladder 47

In Chinese medicine, each of the Five Elements corresponds to one of the five spirits. In a way, the spirit is more fundamental since the qualities and attributes of an Element arise out of the nature of its spirit.

The spirit of Wood is *hun* which occupies the realm of the clouds, lighter than earth but containing enough density to keep it near the earth and not fly away to heaven.

Of all the five spirits, the *hun* is closest to the Western concept of the soul. In fact, the character *hun* is usually translated as Ethereal Soul. The *hun* enters the body after birth and at death it leaves through the top of the head. It then ascends to the stars whereupon 'it reports to the spirits that preside over destiny on the degree to which each of us has cultivated virtue during our lifetime.'[9]

During our life, it is the *hun* which bestows the gifts of Wood upon us. A healthy *hun* allows us to be clear about our purpose in life, find our path, know where we're going and orient ourselves in that direction. It is what helps us to navigate the rapids of life. The *hun* is like the map and compass of our soul.

It is said that during the day the *hun* resides in the eyes to help us to see how we can act in ways that best serve our life purpose.[10] At night when we sleep, it descends to the liver where it organises our dreams. Thus, the *hun* acts as an intermediary between our waking and sleeping states.

If the *hun* is imbalanced, then our sleeping and dreaming may be disrupted. We might suffer from sleep disturbances, sleepwalking, intense dreaming or no dreams at all. In extreme cases we may find it difficult to distinguish between dreams and reality. Out-of-body experiences, near-death experiences, seeing ghosts and spirits are all associations of the *hun*.

The classics say that the liver houses the *hun*,[11] and therefore anything that damages the liver also injures the *hun*. Anger that does not flow freely and gets stuck in the body will damage the liver. It is also easily upset by alcohol and drugs. Marijuana is particularly harmful to the *hun*. While it might seem to endow us with cleverness, creativity and vision when we are intoxicated, over time these very qualities are eroded and we lose both purpose and vitality.

The *hun* can also be injured by psychological scarring. In childhood the *hun* needs psychological support. If a child is severely constrained in his freedom, constantly criticised for his actions or emotionally deprived, the *hun* cannot develop freely. If there is alcoholism or abuse in the home, the development of the *hun* is harmed. In later life too, overwhelming emotional experiences can disturb the *hun*.[12]

The *hun* spirit needs a healthy liver to be invited to stay in the body. Its nature is to wander like a cloud. When its home in our body is unhealthy and uninviting, it will tend to fly away, leaving us bereft of its capacities of clarity, vision and purpose.

The *hun* spirit is what allows us to bring our heavenly nature into earthly form and manifestation. When in balance, it is the source of our dreams and visions, aims and projects, our creativity and ideas, all of which can find expression in physical form in life on earth.

A healthy *hun* is what we need to live a conscious and effective life as a being of spirit in a physical body. This can be supported by the acupoint *Hunmen* – Gate of the Ethereal Soul, the outer *shu* point of the Liver which lies on the Bladder meridian.

Hunmen is a great point for cleansing the liver organ, for treating addictions, and for supporting the healthy functioning of the spirit of Wood. By clearing away stagnation in the Liver Qi, *Hunmen* can resurrect the spirit and activate the core of a person's being.

This point also treats sleep disturbances and insomnia by settling the *hun* spirit during the time of sleep and allowing us to access the wisdom of dreams as they pertain to our life purpose.

When anger and resentment have solidified and been turned inward upon oneself, *Hunmen* can be used to release and mobilise this energy into the service of taking action. Wood that has become rigid and inert can become supple and active, providing the means to express the uniqueness of our individual self in the world.

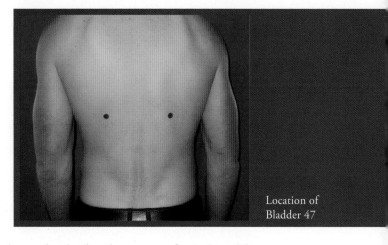

Location of
Bladder 47

Located on the back, about two fingers' width below the bottom of the shoulder blade and 3 cun (four fingers' width) out from the spine. It is level with the space between the 9th and 10th thoracic vertebrae. Use firm, direct pressure.

Combines with LV 3 · LV 14

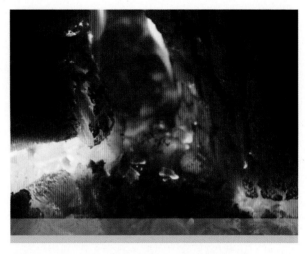

Wood feeds Fire

Xingjian
MOVING
BETWEEN
Liver 2

At the end of spring there is a transitional period of two or three weeks when the energy of Wood is gradually replaced by that of Fire. In the generation or *sheng* cycle, Wood is the mother of Fire. As with all changes of season, this transition is mediated by the Earth Element which arises to smooth the handover.

In humans, it is quite common for the Wood energies to be in excess. This is revealed as a fullness in the Wood pulses. The excess can be calmed by using the sedation point – in this case, the Fire point of a Wood meridian – to move energy around the generation cycle from Wood to Fire.

Xingjian – Moving Between – is an acupoint that achieves this energy transfer. The name refers to the fact that the Liver meridian moves between the first and second toes at the point. But it is also describes its capacity to move Qi between Wood and Fire.

The movement of the Liver Qi is naturally upward. The meridian moves up the insides of the legs, through the groin and abdomen and up into the chest, while a deep pathway continues up through the throat, nose and eyes to the top of the head. But when Liver Qi is in excess, its movement can easily become too rapid and forceful. At its extreme it can become like a raging fire.

Excess Liver energy tends to rise rapidly and often uncontrollably up the body. At the physical level, it can manifest as headaches, dizziness, painful and red eyes, nosebleed, dryness and tightness in the throat, tightness in the chest with difficulty breathing, pain and itching in the genitals, menstrual pain and irregularity, and abdominal distension.

Emotionally, it expresses as anger, frustration and irritability. Anger is the emotion most likely to flare unexpectedly and the most difficult to control. The rapidly rising Liver Qi can produce anger-related symptoms such as a rush of blood to the head, seeing red and flying off the handle. Insomnia can also result.

Moving Between treats all these physical and emotional conditions, quelling the uncontrolled Liver energy by persuading the pent-up energy of Wood to flow smoothly to the Fire Element around the generation cycle.

In the next chapter we will turn our attention to an exploration of the Fire Element. Throughout this summery excursion you will learn some of the important points of the four Fire meridians. Don't forget to bring your hat!

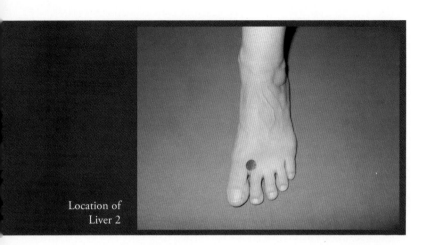

Location of
Liver 2

The point is located just (0.5 cun) above the webbing between the first and second toes. Don't confuse this with Liver 3 which lies further up the foot in a large hollow between the metatarsals. Apply direct pressure.

Combines with LV 3 · LV 14

As spring transitions to summer, there is a qualitative change in the way nature looks and feels. The rapid, uprising, often erratic and unpredictable energy of Wood begins to level out. Nature has gone through its most rapid growth from tender sprout to fully grown plant and the speed of growth begins to slow down. Likewise, the rapid acceleration in the length of the daylight hours also begins to slow. In ourselves, the sense of strongly uprising Qi may be replaced by a feeling of outward expansiveness.

The sun rises quite early now and tries to coax us out of bed earlier than in spring. The days are much longer and the increasing warmth persuades us to shed layers of clothing, to wear lighter and more brightly coloured garments. The temperatures are no longer simply warm but hot. The strength of the sun is noticeably more intense, encouraging us to wear hats and sunscreen. The night comes later, especially if there is daylight saving, encouraging us to stay outdoors and enjoy the lengthening days. Evenings are warm, and there are no longer the cool nights of spring.

In this transition, nature offers us an invitation to come out, to be outdoors more, to be more expansive, both physically, and emotionally. This sense of expansiveness leads naturally to a desire to spend more time with others. The start of summer marks the beginning of the barbeque season, street parties, garage sales and get-togethers of all kinds. Calendars begin to fill up as invitations to social activities surge.

As the energy of Fire begins to replace that of Wood, we may notice more activity in the heart centre, prompting us to seek more human contact and to have more fun in the process.

After spending time exploring the qualities of the Wood Element within you, you have been developing a healthier Wood, healing the gnarled and creaky places in yourself. A healthy Wood Element gives birth to a healthy Fire Element. The work you have done in the spring season will serve as a platform for continued exploration, growth and healing in the summer. As the season transitions to summer and the Fire phase, you will be much better equipped to move into the expansive, loving, heart-oriented Element of Fire.

Ready to fly?

3 Fire

The nature of Fire

The movement of Fire is outwards.

The archetypal image of this Element is the hearth fire. In prehistoric times the human discovery of fire provided a central source of warmth and light, a place for cooking and a means of protection. The tribe gathered around the fire which engendered community and social contact. Even when humans began to settle in villages and live in houses, the hearth fire became the central focus of the home, a place not just for physical heat but for human warmth. Today few people have indoor fires, but campfires and bonfires remain an irresistible draw.

Ultimately, all fire originates from the sun, the biggest, brightest and hottest fire in our world. All fuel for earthly fires originates from the energy of the sun, trapped and stored in the trees.

The various ways that flames and fires behave offer illustrations of the qualities of the Fire Element. As the most yang of the Elements, Fire most exhibits the qualities of yang: hot, bright, expansive, active. Flames dart and leap out in unexpected ways and they go out in all directions. Fire is hot and bright. It can be explosive and bursting like a firework and as overwhelming as a raging forest fire. It can be a fast-burning grassfire that burns itself out quickly, or the slow quiet heat of embers. When fire goes out, it leaves cold grey ashes.

The Chinese character for Fire is *huo*. It represents ascending flames.[1] The flames go out in all directions, a reminder that the fundamental nature of Fire is to move outwards. When I look at this symbol, I see a childlike stick figure of a person running with arms outstretched, fully open to the world.

Resonances of Fire

Season

Summer

The Fire Element is most easily observed in nature as the season of summer. Following the rapid upward growth of spring, nature now reaches outwards to fill as much space as she can. Like a ball tossed in the air which reaches its apogee before descending, summer is the highest peak. Things can grow no further and seem to hang in mid-air for a time, celebrating the fullness of expansion.

Summer is the hottest time of the year because at this time the sun's rays hit the Earth at a steep angle, focusing its energy. Also, the long daylight hours allow the Earth plenty of time to reach warm temperatures. It is the brightest time of the year, with the sun at its highest elevation. Heat and light. Hot and bright. These are intrinsic qualities of summer and of Fire.

When does summer begin? This will depend on your latitude and climate. In temperate climates you can expect to feel the beginnings of summer in early May or early November depending on your hemisphere. This is a month earlier than what is usually considered to be the start of summer, but the first hints of a season are often the most potent in their effects upon us. The transition between spring and summer can be a challenge for some people, an indication of imbalances in Fire.

If you live closer to the equator, summer will come earlier, while if you live closer to the poles, your summer will be later. You can look for the signs of summer within yourself. As the days become warmer, you will wear fewer clothes, and this makes for a feeling of relaxed expansiveness. You will probably find your social calendar gets busier as invitations to summer parties and events jostle with one another for attention. Your view will tend to turn outwards to relationship and community.

Sense
Speech
(Touch)

It is becoming clear that the Fire Element is strongly connected to relationships with others. Perhaps the most common vehicle for humans to connect with one another is through language and speech. The tongue is vital to this process of communication. Speech is therefore the sense of the Fire Element and the tongue its sense organ.[2] This refers not to the tongue as it is used for tasting, but its power to enable speech. Words communicate the feelings of the heart and the content of the mind.

In the West we speak of the five senses of hearing, sight, taste, smell and touch. While the first four of these align neatly with the Elements of Water, Wood, Earth and Metal respectively, it is the sense of speech that is allocated to Fire and touch is not included. Nonetheless, the sense of touch is dependent on the heart-mind as this is responsible for the cognition and organisation of external stimuli sensations.[3]

Touch is certainly in vibrational alignment with the Fire Element. It is a primary component of most relationships, from the handshake to the hug to the tender embrace. It is no accident that all of the Fire meridians travel along the arms and hands, providing a medium for sensing the world and communicating the feelings of the heart.

Summer brings a proliferation of group events, and consequently our communication increases. We tend to be more outgoing and have more opportunities to talk. With the increase in daylight hours, we are likely to stay up later and spend more time interacting. While winter draws our attention inward and spring brings our focus to action,

火

summer invites us to move outwards towards others. The ambient energy of the summer season is supportive of connecting though speech.

When the Fire Element is out of balance, one of the ways is can show up is in speech disorders such as lisping and tongue tie. Many speech disorders such as stuttering are caused by anxiety, stress, shock or trauma. From the Chinese medicine perspective, all of these are manifestations of imbalance in the Heart.

At the other end of the spectrum, Fire imbalance can reveal itself as an overabundance of speech. Not only are there a lot of words but they are delivered at breakneck speed. The speaker bounces around from subject to subject in a chaotic fashion that can be quite exhausting for the listener.

Colour
Red

While the nature of the Fire Element is to proliferate, it might be surprising to consider that its colour, red, is one of the rarer colours in nature. Perhaps it appears so sparingly because it is such an intense colour. Yet its rarity is more than compensated by its vivid visibility. A red sunset captivates us. Flashes of red on birds' wings grab our attention. Red fruits such as strawberries, raspberries and red apples leap out from bushes or trees. Red flowers such as red roses, bottlebrush, poinsettia and hibiscus all stand out strikingly.

Red sports cars are highly noticeable, especially to the police. People with red hair stand out because of their rarity and are stereotypically famous for their fiery nature. Red is the colour of our blood. It is the colour most commonly associated with joy, love, warmth, passion and sexuality, all of which are associations of the Fire Element.

How do you feel when you wear red? If you are always wearing red or hate wearing the colour, it may indicate an imbalance in your Fire. Is there any red in your home? A lot of red can be overpowering, but some red within the house brings Fire into your life. According to *feng shui* principles, it is good to have some red on the Fire wall of a room, the one facing you as you enter.

In Five Element acupuncture diagnosis, the colour red at the sides of the eyes indicates a Fire constitution. However, much more commonly seen is the 'lack of red', a kind of grey, ashen colour that is more usually diagnostic of a Fire type.

Sound Laughing	Whether it is a chuckle, a giggle, a guffaw or a good belly laugh, the sound of Fire is laughter which emanates from the heart. Consistent with the nature of the Element, laughter fizzes up like champagne bubbles rising to the surface and popping, or bursts out unexpectedly and explosively. Laughter is a universal language. While there are thousands of languages and dialects, the way all humans laugh is remarkably similar.

Laughter is used as a signal for being part of a group, indicating acceptance and positive interactions with others. Laughter is often contagious, the laughter of one person provoking laughter in others, creating a feedback loop.

火

Children laugh much more frequently than adults; adulthood is often seen as being a much more serious business. Interestingly, many Fire types look younger than their years, as if the tendency to laughter keeps them more connected to a childlike state.

The laughing voice carries the emotion of joy. A person of Fire constitution has a laughing voice. Sometimes it sounds as if the person is being tickled and is about to burst into laughter. The voice can seem to be rising up, as if lighter than air. These qualities will be present even when the person is not talking about something enjoyable or funny.

Sometimes a Fire person will exhibit 'lack of laugh', a voice which is a flat monotone. The conspicuous absence of laughter suggests that the joy has gone out of their life.

Odour
Scorched

The resonance of odour is the third of the diagnostic tools in determining a person's Constitutional Element. People of a Fire constitution have a scorched odour emanating from their skin. When the person is in good health, this odour is faint and light, like the smell of dry grass in summer. When there is imbalance in the person's health, the odour becomes stronger, like a garment scorched by an iron, or even like burnt toast. The scorched odour is the lightest of the five odours and often the most difficult to catch.

The odour arises from the organs of the Element not doing their job optimally. In this case, the Heart Protector and Triple Heater are the 'organs' that are under stress, producing an imbalance in the heating system of the body and thus the smell of something burning.

Emotion

Joy

The movement of Fire is outwards, so it is natural that its emotion will be expansive. The Fire Element is the highest point of the cycle, so you would expect its emotion to be 'out there'. We speak of bursting with joy and jumping for joy. It is associated with music, dance and parties, all outward-moving expressions of an inner feeling of wellbeing.

Many people, when they come to the Five Element model for the first time, see joy as a positive emotion when compared with anger (Wood) and fear (Water) which are considered negative. Many people feel they would rather be identified as Fire types. But this overlooks the fact that the predominant emotion indicates where someone is most challenged. For the Fire type, there is a fundamental challenge around joy. Either there is a tendency to seek joy most of the time, avoiding thinking or talking about things that bring the mood down, or there is a tendency for joy to be absent, even when it would be appropriate and expected.

The resonance of emotion is the fourth of the diagnostic tools of the Five Element practitioner. When there is a sense of something being not quite right or off note in the area of a person's joy, this will suggest a Fire constitution.

When we are in a situation which engenders happiness or pleasure, we tend to smile and laugh and our voice becomes animated. When the situation changes, these responses also change to be congruent with what is happening. But when the joy continually goes out of control and turns into overexcitement or even hysteria, the practitioner notices an incongruence, or inappropriateness in the joy. Likewise an off note can be observed in a flat joylessness that pervades the person's life.

The Fire Element is unique in that there are four organs and meridians associated with it instead of the usual two. This accords with Fire's burgeoning nature. It is also because the Heart, the most important organ in the body, needs more support and protection from its partner organs. The ancients saw the Heart as the emperor of the kingdom, with the other three organs providing successive levels of defence and protection.

Organs and officials

The Heart is the yin organ of the Fire Element and emperor of the kingdom of the bodymind. 'The Heart holds the office of lord and sovereign. The radiance of the spirits stems from it.'[4] When the sovereign is healthy and rules well, all other organs and officials can do their jobs properly. But when the sovereign is not well, the functioning of the whole court or body is impaired.

The ancient Chinese understood that the Heart governs the Blood and the blood vessels, but more importantly for them, the Heart was a space in which resides the *shen*, that which is both spirit and mind. As the most yang of the spirits, *shen* is the one closest to heaven. Indeed, it is the heavenly light of awareness and consciousness residing in the heart of each one of us.

Other functions of the Heart are that it manifests in the complexion, opens into the tongue, controls the sweat and is affected by excessive joy, hyper-excitement or shock.[5]

The yang organ of Fire is the Small Intestine whose primary task is to absorb nutrition from food and pass the waste on to the large intestine for elimination. An important function of the Small Intestine official, therefore, is that of sorting and choosing between that which is good for us and that which is not. In this way, this yang partner to the Heart acts as its defender and protector by choosing what to let through and what to exclude.

The two other meridians of the Fire Element, the Heart Protector (yin) and Triple Heater (yang), are not organs in the usual sense, but rather functions. The Heart Protector is also known as the Pericardium, named for the double-walled, fluid-filled sac that surrounds the heart like a shock absorber. The Heart Protector defends the Heart, taking the shocks, hurts and betrayals of life in much the same way that a castle's walls protects the keep from invasion.

J.R. Worsley referred to Heart Protector as the Circulation/Sex meridian, reflecting its other significant roles of circulating Blood and expressing the loving feelings associated with sexuality.

The Triple Heater has no corresponding organ or system from the Western medical perspective. The concept that most closely approaches this organ/function is that of homeostasis. This is the capacity of the body to regulate its internal environment and to maintain a stable, relatively constant condition of properties such as temperature and pH.

The Triple Heater is named for the three burning spaces of lower abdomen, upper abdomen and chest. The concept of a burning space comes from the idea of a transforming process like cooking. Indeed, part of the character for the Triple Heater is a chicken roasting over flames.[6] The burners are responsible for receiving, transforming and distributing air and food. These three burning spaces are three interconnecting and mutually supporting chambers. For there to be health and balance, all three must be operating optimally.

The Triple Heater official is responsible for the maintenance of harmony within the empire of the bodymind and in this way protects the Heart. It has a large part to play in the immune system and is sometimes characterised as the customs official protecting the borders of the realm.

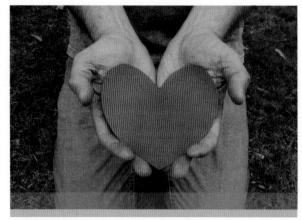

Mind your heart

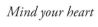

Shenmen
SPIRIT GATE
Heart 7

The Chinese ancients saw the body's organs as having functions far beyond their physiology. They saw the twelve organs as if they were twelve officials in a court, each with a ministerial role and a complex set of functions. They described the functions of these officials much more in terms of mind and spirit than physiology.

From this perspective, the Heart official is akin to an emperor who sits on the throne and holds the kingdom together simply by being himself. When the emperor is wise and moderate and all his ministers are taking care of business, then the kingdom functions harmoniously.

The Heart and its functioning are uniquely essential to life but are also very sensitive to disruption. Because of this, the other three Fire officials (Small Intestine, Heart Protector and Triple Heater) act like an inner cabinet to the emperor. They take on the job of protecting and supporting the Heart, which they do in their various ways, monitoring communications from the Heart to the world and from the world back to the Heart.

The spirit of the Heart is *shen*. One modern authority, Giovanni Maciocia, translates *shen* as mind;[7] indeed, the ancients saw no distinction between heart and mind, unlike the usual Western view that mind is equivalent to brain function.

When the heart-mind is settled and protected, the *shen* resides there quietly. However, *shen* is easily disturbed by shock and trauma which can cause it to fly away like a flock of startled birds. When the *shen* leaves the Heart, the connection with spirit is lost and the person may feel apathetic, depressed and separated from themselves and the world. Others may see emptiness, vacancy and lifelessness in their eyes.

On the other hand, disturbance to the *shen* can result in hyper-excitement, a kind of false joy that appears ungrounded and unreal. Insomnia, restless activity, uncontrolled speech and even mania can be some of the manifestations of such disturbance to the Heart.

In choosing points to treat the Heart, we must be very careful to respect its delicate sensitivity. Some acupuncturists do not even use needles on the Heart meridian, preferring instead to treat it indirectly through Heart Protector. Heart must be treated gently, treasured and honoured like an infant king.

One point that is safe to use is *Shenmen* – Spirit Gate. It is the gateway into the innermost chamber of the Heart. At the same time, it provides a gateway through which the Heart can express itself in the world. As the source point of the Heart meridian, it treats the organ directly, strengthening and stabilising it. The point will balance the Qi whether it is deficient or excess.

Shenmen soothes the mind and spirit, easing anxiety, sadness, depression and mania. It helps to mend a broken heart. It calms the physical heart, treating such conditions as pounding, palpitations and arrhythmia. *Shenmen* assists with memory and mental capacity; it helps with conditions of speech and the tongue, including excessive speech; and it helps when there is insomnia and restless sleep, calming the heart and mind to allow for peaceful rest.

In the West we refer to the eyes as the windows of the soul. The perspective of Chinese medicine is that the eyes are windows into the heart-mind. The quality of the *shen* is seen in the eyes. When the *shen* is healthy, the eyes are alive with a 'thereness' that makes intimate contact with the world, while at the same time the person is in contact with himself. Spirit Gate helps us to move towards this way of being in the world.

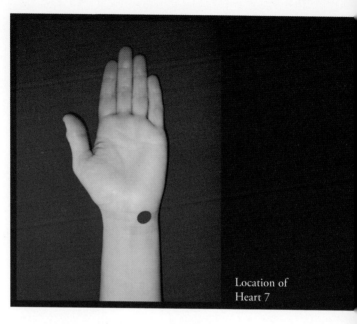

Location of
Heart 7

The point lies on the inner wrist crease, towards the ulnar (little finger) side and about one-fifth of the distance across the wrist. Feel for a hollow at the base of the pisiform bone. Apply gentle, direct pressure. Tune into yourself as you do this. Treat it as a little meditation on your heart.

Combines with SI 7 · HP 7 · CV 17

Choosing wisely

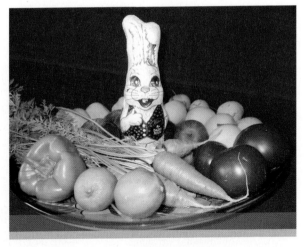

Zhizheng
BRANCH OF
THE UPRIGHT
Small Intestine 7

The Heart is protected by three ministers or officials of the Fire Element. The Small Intestine official, sometimes referred to as the Sorter, is the minister who is closest to the sovereign Heart. His job description includes the functions of personal assistant, liaison officer, food taster, adviser and friend. Just as the organ of small intestine sorts the pure from the impure in the food we eat, so too the Small Intestine official is responsible for sorting out what is good for the Heart and what is not. This sorting includes the transformation of food and the absorption of nutrients, but also operates more widely at the level of mind and spirit.

Small Intestine is the paired partner of the Heart. It is yang to the Heart's yin. This official listens attentively to the needs of the Heart and is in constant, direct contact with it. This close attention facilitates the communication from the Heart to the outside world and from the world back to the Heart.

An imbalance in Small Intestine can cause a breakdown in the attentiveness to the Heart's needs. This might result in making poor food choices, taking in food that is not good for the body. It may also extend to choosing relationships that are harmful or situations that are toxic, and failing to engage in activities that nourish the spirit. In our busy modern world we have so many choices to make, so much information to filter and sort, that the Small Intestine official can become overwhelmed and fail to adequately protect his friend, the king.

When the Small Intestine is not listening to the Heart, it tends also not to listen to the world. There can be confusion in communicating with others, misunderstanding what others are saying and being misunderstood by them.

A point to support the healthy relationship between Small Intestine and Heart is *Zhizheng* – Branch of the Upright. This is the *luo*-connecting point of the meridian which supports balance between the yin and yang meridians. The upright referred to here is the Heart itself, while the branch is the connecting channel.

Zhizheng helps to resolve ambivalence and confusion by conveying faithfully the intent of the Heart. It calms and balances the Heart when its spirit (*shen*), is disrupted by restlessness, fluctuating moods, fright, anxiety, depression or mania.

At the physical level, Branch of the Upright is used to treat problems of the forearm and elbow, painful fingers and difficulty gripping. As with most Small Intestine points, it treats problems in the shoulder and neck through which the meridian passes. It also reduces fever, visual dizziness and blurred vision.

If you have trouble sorting the sheep from the goats, get confused about the choices in your life, or have lost touch with what your heart is telling you, *Zhizheng* can help restore connection with the purity of your Heart.

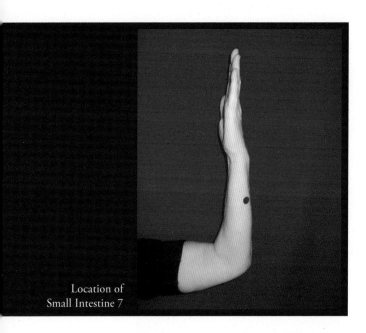

Location of
Small Intestine 7

The point is on the ulnar (little finger) side of the forearm, five-twelfths of the distance between the wrist and the elbow (5 cun). Locate with your arm bent as shown. The point lies in the hollow between the ulna bone and the muscle next to it on the front of the arm (carpi ulnaris). Use direct pressure.

Combines with H 7 · SI 3 · SI 10

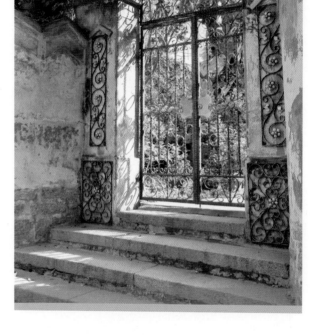

The second of the three officials guarding the emperor Heart is the Heart Protector. It acts as a defensive wall around the Heart, protecting it from shock and hurt in the way that the double-walled sac of the pericardium protects the organ of the heart.

Neiguan – Inner Frontier Gate – is a significant point on the Heart Protector meridian and one of the most important of all the acupoints. Its

Neiguan
INNER
FRONTIER GATE
Heart Protector 6

hallmark is its capacity to bring steadiness to the bodymind. It steadies the heart, the circulation, the stomach, the mind and the emotions.

To begin with, *Neiguan* is one of the strongest points influencing the chest and the chest cavity. It is the *luo*-connecting point of the Heart Protector, connecting to its partner the Triple Heater. But this connection with the Triple Heater is not at the forearm where the point is located but in the chest. This point therefore exerts a profound influence over the Heart and Lungs and promotes the circulation of Qi and Blood in all three Burners.

Neiguan is also the master point of the *Yin Wei Mai* (Yin Linking Vessel) which connects all yin meridians and influences the chest and Heart. It treats chest pain, pain in the ribs, palpitations, arrhythmia and hypertension. It relaxes the coronary arteries and is known to have a general analgesic effect.

As an important Fire point, it regulates the Fire Element, balancing it whether it is raging out of control or burning too low. It is particularly known for heat conditions such as fevers, hot skin, cracked tongue and painful urination.

At the emotional level, the point has a steadying influence on the Heart, calming the spirit, clearing the brain and brightening the mental outlook when joylessness has pervaded the Heart Protector. It treats a wide range of emotional disorders such as irritability, anxiety, depression, mania, fear, fright and sadness. By steadying the Heart and the *shen*, it treats insomnia.

As the name implies, Inner Frontier Gate integrates the inner and outer. It regulates the connection between the Heart and the outer world, facilitating communication between the two. The Heart Protector protects the Heart by closing when appropriate in hurtful situations and opening to connect emotionally in loving relationships. Nowhere is this function seen more clearly than at Inner Frontier Gate. When healthy, it is a gate that swings easily on its hinges.

Where there has been pain, shock, betrayal and trauma to the Heart, *Neiguan* has the capacity to heal old wounds. A person suffering post-traumatic stress disorder (PTSD) continually re-experiences the initial trauma, whether from physical accident, frightening situations or physical or sexual abuse. All of these traumas are absorbed by the Heart Protector and can be treated at this point.

The other major area in which *Neiguan*'s steadying influence is felt, is the Stomach. It is a significant point for the Stomach and the go-to point for nausea and vomiting due to its connection with the Triple Heater and the Lower Burner. The point steadies the Stomach by treating all kinds of nausea including seasickness or other motion sickness, morning sickness in pregnancy and nausea experienced during chemotherapy. Its effectiveness for nausea has been well documented as there have been more scientific studies of *Neiguan* than any other acupoint.

When you find that your heart, mind or stomach are all at sea, try holding *Neiguan* to steady your ship.

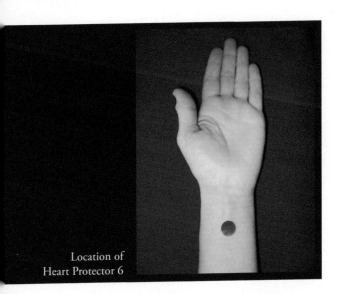

Location of
Heart Protector 6

The point lies on the front of the forearm between the ulna and radius bones, 2 cun (approximately three fingers' width) above the inner wrist crease. Use moderate, direct pressure.

Combines with TH 5 · HP 7 · HP 8 · CV 17 · SP 4 · SP 16 · LV 14

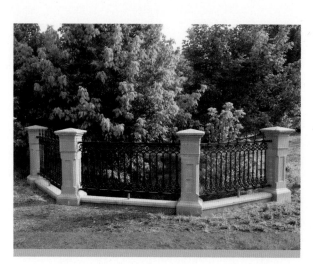

Guarding the frontier

The third of the officials that protect the Heart is the Triple Heater. It is the outermost of the Fire officials, concerned with protecting the borders of the kingdom. This relates to protection of the exterior of the body and to negotiating social and societal relationships.

Waiguan
OUTER
FRONTIER GATE
Triple Heater 5

At the physical level, the Triple Heater maintains homeostasis in the body. In particular, it is the thermostat, keeping the body's temperature in the Goldilocks zone, neither too hot nor too cold. It regulates conditions in the three burning spaces (lower abdomen, upper abdomen and chest) for which it is named, and maintains the crucial balance between Fire (yang) and Water (yin). It plays a role in the immune system, keeping harmony among all other officials, coordinating the functions of all the organs and ensuring harmonious interaction between them.

At the psycho-emotional level, Triple Heater manages social relationships, deciding who in the world it is safe to befriend and who can be trusted to enter the kingdom of the Heart. In this sense, it sets boundaries, restricting the entry of people who may harm us and guiding our own appropriate social behaviour. Here, Triple Heater works closely with Heart Protector.

When Triple Heater falls out of balance, there can be disruption to the heating system of the body, causing one to feel very hot or very cold, and sometimes both in rapid succession. A person might hate the winter and love the summer, or vice versa. At an emotional level, it can make for difficulty in distinguishing between social and intimate relationships, falling in love quickly and repeatedly, behaving in socially inappropriate ways, even becoming an exhibitionist.

The point *Waiguan* – Outer Frontier Gate – is the most important point on the Triple Heater meridian. It is an effective one for keeping balance and harmony between the Heart and the wider world, resolving conflicts between the inner and outer. As the *luo*-connecting point of the channel, it connects to the Heart Protector meridian through HP 6 and is often used with it to balance the channel with its yin partner.

Another of its roles is as the master point of the *Yang Wei Mai* (Yang Linking Vessel) which rules the exterior of the whole body and connects all of the yang meridians. Therefore, it can be used for all external pathogenic invasions from wind, cold, heat and damp, as well as fever and many types of headaches.

Waiguan treats ear disorders including tinnitus, deafness, earache and itching ears. It is also good for pain and stiffness of the neck, shoulder, elbow, arm and hand.

Forearm yourself against external invasion from disease and guard your heart from harmful influences by strengthening the guard at the Outer Frontier Gate.

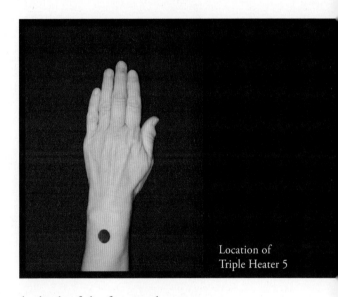

Location of
Triple Heater 5

The point lies on the back of the forearm between the ulna and radius bones, 2 cun (approximately three fingers' width) above the wrist where it bends when flexed. Use moderate, direct pressure.

Combines with HP 6 · SI 10 · CV 17 ·
GB 20 · GB 21 · GB 41 · GV 16

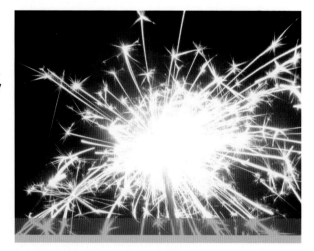

Light my fire!

Laogong
PALACE OF
WEARINESS
Heart Protector 8

As a teenager, I well remember getting very excited at hearing The Doors song 'Light My Fire'. It literally lit me up, raising energy in joyful, expansive, rippling shivers. I just listened to the song again on YouTube and it still makes me tingle. Music has this capacity to stir the heart, to excite, to expand. So too does love, whether it is a love of chocolate, passion for a vocation or hobby, or desire for another person.

When our Fire Element is balanced, we have easy access to these qualities of joy, love, desire and passion. But when Fire is out of balance, there can be flatness, dullness, lack of joy and a reduced interest in intimacy. On the other hand, when the imbalance manifests as Fire out of control, there can be hyper-excitement, mania, babbling speech and feverish behaviour.

Laogong – Palace of Weariness – is the Fire point on the Heart Protector meridian and is a power point for balancing the Fire Element. It lies near the middle of the palm and is considered to be a minor chakra.[8] If you hold your palms facing each other, you will probably feel a sensation of warmth, tingling, pressure or pulsing. You are activating the Qi at these points. Those who do healing work will often use this point through which to channel healing energy to another person.

When you hold this point on yourself or another, it stirs the Fire in the way you might rake a dying fire into life. It activates and opens the emotional heart. When a person feels no joy in their life, feels flat and depressed, low in spirit and weary of life, then Palace of Weariness can restore vitality, vigour and love for life. It can encourage those who have had their heart broken, crushed or betrayed to enter anew into relationships. It can also support someone whose heart is tender and sensitive, who wears their heart on their sleeve or whose heart needs protection.

At the other extreme, this point can calm an overactive Heart and quiet a restless mind. For those who suffer from bipolar symptoms, alternating between manic and depressed phases, this is a balancing point. It can also help those who are addicted to falling in love or who fall quickly in and out of love.

Laogong also treats a range of physical conditions that relate to the Fire Element including cardiac pain, epilepsy, palpitations, arrhythmia, fever, nosebleed, mouth and tongue ulcers, and cold hands.

Next time you feel you need help to follow Jim Morrison's advice to set the night on fire, come on, baby, hold *Laogong*.

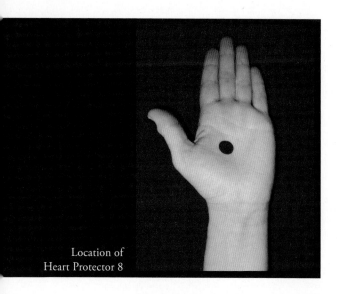

Location of
Heart Protector 8

The point is located in the palm of the hand, in the depression between the second and third metacarpals. If you make a fist, the point is where the tip of the middle finger touches the palm. Use moderate, direct pressure.

Combines with HP 6 · HP 7 · CV 17

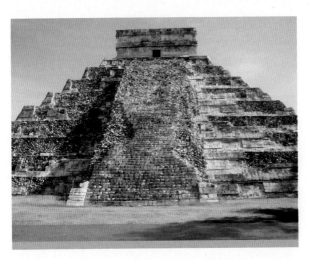

Stairway to heaven

This is not a reference to the infamous Led Zeppelin classic, much beloved by air guitarists, but a poetic description of the spinal column. Stairway to Heaven is one of the names given to a point at the base of the coccyx, the first point of the *Du Mai* (Governing Vessel) whose pathway travels up the length of the spine and over the head. *Houxi*, a powerful point of the Small Intestine meridian, is also the master point of the Governing Vessel and so benefits any conditions along this pathway. This includes pain or misalignment of any of the vertebrae of the back and neck. There is an acupoint at almost every vertebral junction, and these can be held in combination with SI 3 for treatment of spinal problems.

In its capacity as master point of the Governing Vessel, *Houxi* also helps with problems of the lumbar region and the kidneys. It treats occipital (back) and vertex (top) headaches as well as neck pain, chills or fever caused by wind. The point

Houxi
BACK STREAM
Small Intestine 3

invigorates mental functioning, allowing for greater clarity of thought.

Back Stream also powerfully affects the channel of Small Intestine and is particularly effective in treating elbow, upper back and shoulder pain as well as neck pain and stiffness, difficulty turning the head, and neck pain that is aggravated by nodding. It treats conditions of the sensory orifices: tinnitus, deafness, redness and swelling of the eyes and nosebleed. It treats conditions of the finger joints, particularly the little and ring fingers.

Since Small Intestine exerts an influence over its partner, the Heart, *Houxi* can treat cardiac pain and palpitations, settle the *shen*, ease agitation and insomnia. It is good for treating epilepsy and bipolar disorder, which are disturbances of the *shen*. It can clear heat from the body.

Houxi is the Wood point of the Small Intestine meridian and so balances the qualities of Wood within the Fire. The forthright, direct, uprising energy of Wood fuels the flourishing and maturing of our plans and projects. The point can give a person backbone and the strength to make difficult choices.

At the physical level, *Houxi* benefits the tendons and ligaments which enable us to move into action, while psychologically it brings clarity and determination to the process of choosing and deciding how to negotiate the stairways of life.

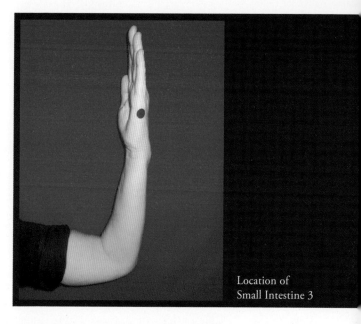

Location of
Small Intestine 3

On the side of the hand at the base of the little
finger. If you make a loose fist, the point can be
found in a sizeable depression between the finger
and the fifth metacarpal bone.

Combines with SI 10 · H 7 · BL 62 ·
GV 4 · GV 16 · any point on the spine

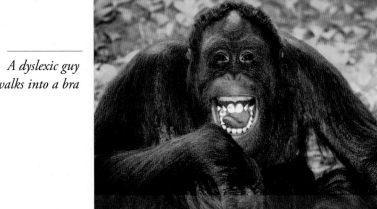

A dyslexic guy walks into a bra

Daling
GREAT MOUND
Heart Protector 7

I'm a sucker for the snappy one liner and this one from George Carlin is a cracker. And this is just the tip of the funny bone. From puns to pies in the face, the parrot sketch to shaggy dog stories, from stand-up to the Groucho put-down, there are countless things that make us giggle, snicker, titter, chuckle and plain laugh out loud.

A good sense of humour is a great asset and support on the rocky road of life. Dating sites are full of people looking for a partner with a GSOH, presumably someone who will laugh at their jokes.

Laughter is not confined to the arena of joke-telling. Experiencing something unexpected can produce laughter. We can laugh spontaneously, feeling the joy of simply being alive. Laughter is the sound of joy bubbling out of the heart.

There are medical benefits too. Neurophysiology indicates that laughter is linked with the activation of the prefrontal cortex, the part of the brain that produces endorphins.[9] The old adage that laughter is the best medicine is being borne out by modern science.

There are many Fire points that can help us to access this lighter side of life. It is interesting to note that the first point of the Heart meridian lies tucked in the armpit, one of the classic places to be tickled. Another is Heart Protector 8 in the palm of the hand. I once had a series of acupuncture treatments that included this point and every time it was needled I went into fits of giggling that had my acupuncturist and me in stitches.

Another important point that can help to access the laughter of the Heart and its many other qualities is the Heart Protector point *Daling* – Great Mound. When there is lack of joy or deep sadness, this point is helpful, for it calms the *shen*, spirit of the Heart. Indeed, it is a good point for any emotional stress including anxiety, hysteria, grief, fear, fright and panic. When there is a feeling of vulnerability or insecurity, or a person is suffering relationship trauma, *Daling* is called for.

At the physical level, Great Mound regulates the Heart and relaxes the chest. It treats palpitations caused by fright, intercostal pain, eczema and other skin conditions arising from heat. It settles the stomach and intestines. Locally it can treat tendinitis and carpal tunnel syndrome.

The classic text *The Spiritual Pivot* described the Heart Protector as the channel that pertains to the Heart, so *Daling* was originally indicated as the source point of the Heart rather than *Shenmen*, Heart 7.[10] Therefore, this is a powerful portal to the Heart and its qualities of joy, contentment, radiance, equanimity, love and laughter.

By the way, did you hear the one about…?

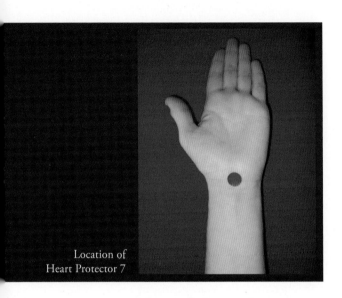

Location of
Heart Protector 7

The point lies in the very centre of the anterior (front) wrist crease. It lies between the tendons of palmaris longus and flexor carpi radialis. Use gentle, direct pressure.

Combines with HP 6 · HP 8 · H7 · CV 17

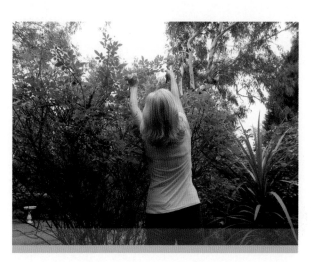

Shoulder problems are common in the treatment room. Shoulders get a lot of work and are easily imbalanced because of the large number of muscles that are involved in their movement. The scapula or shoulder blade is the foundation of the shoulder girdle. It has one articulating joint, the acromioclavicular (AC) joint at the point of the shoulder. Otherwise, its position is entirely governed by the degree of strength and suppleness of the 17 muscles that attach to it.

A key point in this area is *Naoshu* – Upper Arm Shu. I have a certain fondness for this point because it was one of the points I learned in my first acupressure class. It forms part of a five-step neck and shoulder release that I still use in the treatment room and teach in my classes.[11]

I was reminded recently of the power of this point when I spent 15 minutes working on someone at a farmers' market in a massage chair. The man was a fruit grower who spent a lot of time

Naoshu
UPPER ARM SHU
Small Intestine 10

reaching above his head to pick fruit. His right shoulder had seized up, causing such pain that he needed large doses of painkillers to control it. His right arm was virtually immobilised. I found that the Qi at *Naoshu* was seriously blocked, but after a full five minutes of pressure, the point popped open and Qi began to flow through the shoulder. The pain was almost gone and freedom of movement was restored.

One reason this point is so powerful is that it lies on two of the Extraordinary Vessels, the *Yang Wei Mai* (Yang Linking Vessel) and the *Yang Qiao Mai* (Yang Motility Vessel). In addition, it is a meeting point with the Bladder meridian. Because it is such a nexus, there are many reasons why it can become blocked, but it also means that there are more ways that it can be useful. It is very potent when used in combination with TH 5, the master point of the Yang Linking Vessel.

Naoshu treats a wide range of shoulder problems including pain, stiffness, swelling and weakness of the shoulder. It benefits where there is restricted movement including inability to raise the arm. It also helps to relieve the condition known as adhesive capsulitis (frozen shoulder).

As with many Small Intestine points, *Naoshu* affects the length of the channel, and so treats tinnitus and deafness. It also treats fever and excessive underarm perspiration, and helps to eliminate toxins from the body.

If you have the weight of the world on your shoulders, use *Naoshu* to help shrug it off.

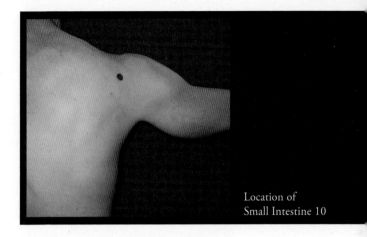

Location of
Small Intestine 10

The point lies in a depression below the spine of the scapula and above the posterior crease of the armpit. With the arm by the side, draw up the channel between the arm and the shoulder blade until you are just below the bone of the scapular spine. If you then raise your arm above your head, the depression becomes much more obvious. Use firm angled pressure that is superior (upwards) and medial (towards the shoulder blade).

Combines with TH 5 . SI 3 . SI 7

All you need is love

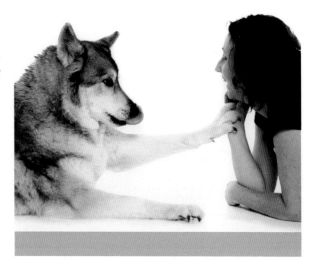

Shanzhong
WITHIN THE
BREAST
Conception Vessel 17

Perhaps more words have been written and spoken about love than any other subject. Certainly, it is a major focus in books, movies and popular music. There is no simple definition of love because it has different meanings in different contexts. There are many kinds of love.

We can say we love certain foods such as ice cream or chocolate, we love our hobbies or our work, we love our pets, we love our neighbours, we love our family, we love our partner, we love the earth, we love God.

Whichever culture or system you look at, there seems to be universal agreement that love is associated with the heart. Whatever kind of love we are talking about, it is a state that is perceived by and expressed through the heart centre. Love is often experienced as a warm or expansive feeling in the chest. This is a direct experience of the fact that the heart is the primary organ of the Fire Element. The extent to which we are able to feel love, receive love, give love or express love will indicate the health of our Fire.

The Fire point that lies in the very centre of the chest is *Shanzhong* – Within the Breast. While it lies on the *Ren Mai* (Conception Vessel), it is the *mu* or alarm point for the Heart Protector. This is where the *shen*, the spirit of the Heart, resides. It coincides with the heart chakra or heart centre and is the place where we most feel our heart feelings. It is where we feel the pleasurably warm, glowing feeling when we fall in love and also where the pain is felt when our heart is broken.

Shanzhong is a point that activates the *shen*, the spirit of the Heart. It facilitates the communication of feelings from the Heart to the outside and helps to settle the spirit when the person has been exhausted or betrayed by relationships. When the heart has gone cold, it opens the Heart Protector to new possibilities of engagement with others.

At the physical level, this point strongly activates Qi in the chest, affecting both heart and lungs. It treats tightness in the chest, chronic cough and shortness of breath. Because it quells rebellious Qi in the middle burner, it aids heartburn and acid reflux. It also facilitates lactation and treats mastitis.

While this point won't guarantee you'll find the love of your life, it can help you to open the conduit for communication of feelings and for the giving and receiving of love.

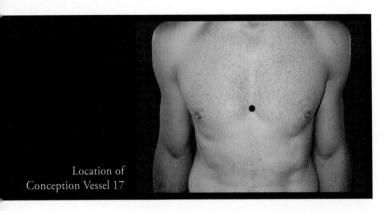

Location of
Conception Vessel 17

The point is in the centre of the sternum in a shallow hollow. On men it lies between the nipples. It is at the level of the fourth intercostal space which is most accurately located by counting down four rib spaces from the underside of the clavicle. The point can be held with gentle, direct finger pressure, or more gently still by placing the palm on or over the point.

Combines with H 7 · HP 6 · HP 7 · HP 8 · TH 5

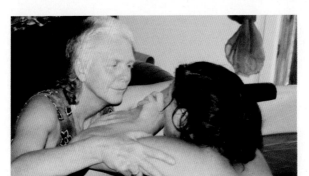

Healing trauma

It is the nature of being human that we are vulnerable. We inhabit fragile bodies and have delicate feelings. We are sensitive to many external stimuli from physical objects, and from what other people do and say to us. We are influenced, even if we don't know it, by the thoughts and feelings of others. It is this vulnerability that gives us the capacity for deep contact with others and the world. But it also means that we are easily hurt.

Gaohuangshu
RICH FOR
THE VITALS
Bladder 43

Babies are born totally vulnerable. It is one reason they are so adorable. But soon the child develops a protective shell to shield her from the slings and arrows of life in the human realm. When these traumas of life are outrageous, egregious, and they penetrate the shell, it is the Heart Protector that absorbs the shock so as to protect the Heart. When the insults to the Heart are great, the Heart Protector is deeply injured. Therefore, healing trauma requires healing the Heart Protector.

One of the best points for working with trauma of all kinds is the outer *shu* point of the Heart Protector, *Gaohuangshu* – Rich for the Vitals, which lies between the shoulder blades and behind the heart.

This point exerts a strong influence over the official of the Heart Protector, especially at emotional and psychological levels. However, the point name itself refers to the *Gaohuang*, a region in the chest, whose influence is much wider and deeper than that of the Heart Protector alone.

The *Gaohuang*, or Vital Region, is an area in the chest about four body inches in diameter, lying between the centre and base of the sternum, and extending laterally to the pathways of the Kidney meridian.

When there is illness that is caused by deep heartbreak, betrayal, abuse, shame or isolation, this vital region is deeply impacted and the effects go deep into our being. Jarrett sees this as a place where deep karmic issues and conflicts reside, and where dark family secrets live.[12] Chronic or incurable disease is said to lodge here.

Classical texts observe that *Gaohuangshu* deeply nourishes and calms the Heart as well as Kidney and Spleen. The action of this point was considered so great that it was said to strengthen the original Qi and treat every kind of deficiency. Sun Si-miao, the famous 7th-century physician, went so far as to say that there is no disorder it cannot treat.[13]

Gaohuangshu is a great tonic point for the physical body, treating exhaustion and general deficiency, increasing stamina and supporting all the organs. It brings warmth and strength and increases blood circulation.

At the emotional level, the point brings warmth when a person is emotionally cold and shut down. It helps to dispel depression and mental negativity. When someone has little capacity for intimacy and humour because they are too depleted or vulnerable, this point lifts the spirit.

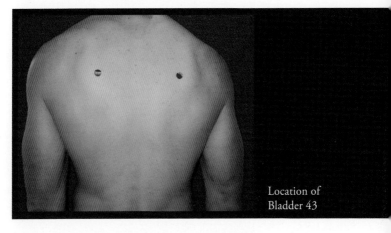

Location of
Bladder 43

Gaohuangshu is located between the shoulder blades, 3 cun lateral to the midline, at the level of the junction of T4 and T5 and at the medial border of the scapula. It is approximately halfway down the scapula. Use firm, direct pressure. To treat yourself, lie on a tennis ball or other object that presses into the point. Arrange the pressure so you can be as relaxed as possible. Having someone you trust hold this point can be very healing.

Combines with HP 7 · H 7 · HP 8 · CV 17

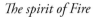

The spirit of Fire

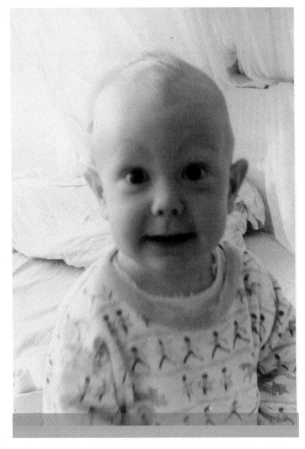

Shentang
SPIRIT HALL
Bladder 44

Shen is the spirit of the Fire Element. As the most yang of the spirits, it is the one closest to heaven. It is the heavenly light of awareness and consciousness residing in the heart of each one of us. When the heart is healthy, it provides a place for the *shen* to rest. But when the heart is unhealthy, disturbed and unsettled, the *shen* flies away like a flock of birds startled by a commotion.

In the classical literature, *shen* is used in two ways. In the first, it refers collectively to all five spirits (*wu shen*), five individual aspects of consciousness, each expressing the nature of its corresponding Element. In the second sense, *shen* refers particularly to the spirit of the Fire Element. This spirit is responsible for thought, feeling, emotions, perceptions and cognition. The heart and the mind are so inextricably linked that the *shen* of the Heart is often translated as mind or heart-mind. The *shen* of Fire resides in the Heart during our lifetime; upon our death, the spirit returns to the heavenly realm where it originated.

The *shen* is not directly visible, but it is reflected in a person's eyes as a sparkle, a point of contact, a 'thereness'. This inner radiance, called *shen ming*, is what gives each person his personal uniqueness. It is that which makes each of us like no other.

The *shen* is reflected also in a settled mind and clear thinking. When the *shen* is disturbed, has flown away, the eyes become dull and there is a sense that the person is not quite there. Shock, trauma and abuse are common reasons for the *shen* to fly. People who have experienced war, imprisonment or torture, or refugees who are fleeing persecution are often likely to have *shen* disturbance and therefore Heart imbalance.

The spirit of the Heart is responsible for settled sleep and settled emotions, and cognitive functions such as concentration, short-term memory and the ability to think clearly. *Shen* disturbance can therefore appear as difficulty getting to sleep, dream disturbance, volatile emotions, anxiety, panic, depression and feelings of rejection. Since *shen* is the mind of the heart, any disturbance will result in disturbances of the mind. Indeed, all mental illness can be viewed as an imbalance in the *shen*.

A healthy and balanced Heart *shen* enables the capacity to form and maintain healthy and meaningful relationships. Heart boundaries are clear but also able to adapt appropriately to different relationships. Conversely, emotional problems that stem from relationships, such as abandonment and betrayal, weaken the Heart and hurt the *shen*.

What does *shen* look like when it is in perfect balance? Such a person is settled, calm and not easily distracted. She sleeps peacefully, undisturbed by dreams. She has an inner light that infuses her with a glow that can be seen in the eyes. She makes eye contact that shows her depth. Her speech is coherent, reflecting a balanced mind. The way she lives her life is congruent with who she is as a person. She gives and receives love with ease. In a way she lives a life of love. She may well be intuitive, her consciousness in open communication with universal consciousness.

A point that strongly influences the *shen* is *Shentang* – Spirit Hall. It is the outer *shu* point of the Heart and lies on the Bladder meridian. *Shentang* makes direct contact with the heart-mind and has the capacity to restore the *shen* to the Heart. It brings us back to the centre of who we are in our uniqueness as a drop of the Tao

When the *shen* is disturbed and there is anxiety, depression or heartbreak, or when we are resigned, in a state of shock or without the capacity to act, then Spirit Hall can restore the spirit and encourage participation once more in the richness of life.

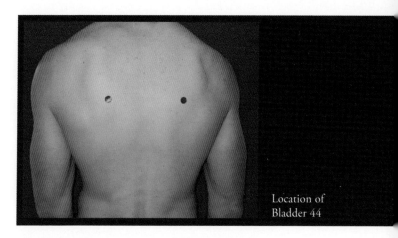

Location of
Bladder 44

Shentang is located between the shoulder blades. It is 3 cun lateral to the midline at the level of the junction of T5 and T6 and at the medial border of the scapula. This point is best held by someone else using firm, direct pressure. To treat yourself, lie on a tennis ball or golf ball pressing into this point. It is best if you can be relaxed so that you can tune into the subtle influences that this point can bring.

Combines with H 7 · HP 7 · CV 17

Transition from Fire to Earth

There comes a day when summer feels as if it has finally burnt itself out. It is reminiscent of a boisterous party which has talked and laughed and danced away the night but finally runs out of energy and needs to take a rest. Nature's riotous summer foliage has reached its peak and now begins to droop. The sun's angle begins to drop and its heat is no longer intense. The light is softer, more golden. The days become noticeably shorter. Overall, there is a sense of lessening and decreasing. The summer holiday and party season is over. School goes back.

For some this is a time of sadness that the great summer party is over for another year. For those who love the summer heat, the end of the warmest season can engender a longing for it to continue. Some even fear the coming cold. There may be a feeling of poignancy at its ending. For those who find the high temperatures unbearable, there is a relief that the intense heat is finally over.

Because the season of late summer is itself a transition, the transitions from summer to late summer and from late summer to autumn happen quickly over the space of a few weeks. As with all transitions, there can be a going back and forth between the seasons. In some climates the hottest days are at this time of year, as if the summer is having one last dance at the party, one last drink for the road.

Whatever your feelings about heat and summer, whether you love it and don't want it to end, or you hate it and can't wait for it to leave, or you are somewhere in between, take time to be as fully present as you can with the changes that are happening both around you and within you. This transition will come again in other years, but never again in quite the way it is this year. This is a unique moment in your life and in the life of the planet. Just be. Right here.

Now.

4 Earth

The importance of Earth is reflected in the many
meanings of the word. Earth is one of the Five
Elements. It is also the name of the planet, our
home in space. It describes the soil which grows
the food that sustains us. And it is the supportive
ground upon which we stand and move.

All of the other Elements have a direction of
movement. Wood is upwards, Fire is outwards,
Metal is downwards and Water is inwards. Rather
than having a direction of movement, Earth acts
as an axis, fulcrum or centre around which all the
other Elements move.

Earth energy is therefore neutral and is not classified as either yin or yang. It is the place of balance. It is the hub of the wheel from which spokes radiate, the point of reference to which other things are oriented. This notion of centrality is seen physically in the way the Earth organs of Stomach and Spleen are central to digestion, and psycho-emotionally in the way Earth energy likes to mediate and bring people together.

Earth energy is also seen in the principle of gravity. Gravity is the force that attracts a body to the centre of the Earth. Whatever is thrown into the air returns to Earth, comes back to centre. It is Earth's gravity that gives us weight and keeps us grounded.

Earth creates shape, form and holding. It provides the banks that give shape and form to rivers and lakes. It provides stable ground on which to build. It supports our every step.

The Chinese character for Earth is *tu*. The top horizontal line represents the surface of the soil while the bottom line represents the subsoil or bedrock. The vertical line represents all that is produced by the earth. The character therefore conveys two significant qualities of Earth, those of nourishment and stability.[1]

The Earth Element has its own season of late summer and is also the facilitator of transitions between the seasons. The *Neijing* says that Earth energy is at its height in late summer.[2] But it also states that Earth's season is the last 18 days of each season and that it does not have a distinct season of its own.[3] From this we understand that Earth energy is evident four times a year at the changing of the four seasons, but most particularly at the end of the summer.

The late summer is the harvest time, Keats' season of 'mellow fruitfulness'[4] when nature takes a well-earned rest from producing and lies about in the warm fields, lazily listening to the humming of bees. The last fruit hangs heavy and round on the trees, oozing and dripping ripeness.

Many annual plants are looking droopy, drying out and going to seed. While the temperatures are still warm, the sting has gone out of the sun, whose angle in the sky begins to dip. Days shorten noticeably and early sunsets allow for cooler evenings.

When does late summer begin? This will vary depending on your location. The Chinese almanac, the Tong Shu, puts this transition in late July and early August (late January and early February in the southern hemisphere). Warmer climates may feel the change later. Overall, there is a sense of a decrease in nature, a lowering of intensity, a softening and rounding. You may feel these qualities within yourself.

Resonances
of Earth

Season
Late summer
and transitions

Earth energy appears in the late summer, but also in the late autumn, late winter and late spring, arising at these times to mediate between the differing qualities of the four seasons. The Chinese word *doyo* describes this time of transition. In the way that 'twilight' and 'dusk' refer to the transition between day and night, the word *doyo* denotes each of the four seasonal transitions.

Earth is most specifically awarded the place between Fire and Metal because the qualities of nurturance, abundance, fullness and ripeness align it naturally to the time of harvest, the season of nature's maturing.

The ease with which you are able to flow with the transitions between seasons will offer insights into the health and stability of the Earth Element within you.

Sense

Taste

One of the newborn baby's first experiences is of the taste of mother's milk. At a very early stage in life, taste becomes associated with mother's comfort, support and love. In later life this sense can become strongly linked to deriving comfort from food.

The sense of taste is closely related to the stomach because it is the taste buds which identify foods that are good for us to eat. The mouth, lips, oesophagus and stomach are all part of the system that identifies, chooses and ingests food. The same receptors identify things that are not good for us; for example, many poisonous foods are bitter in flavour.

The sensation of taste, or gustation, originates in the taste buds, but also includes the sense of smell in rounding out the experience of flavour. The taste buds are taste receptor cells which identify the various flavours from food dissolved in saliva. There are five flavours which correspond to the Five Elements: salty (Water), sour (Wood), bitter (Fire), sweet (Earth) and pungent or savoury (Metal).

Craving for or aversion to a particular flavour can indicate an imbalance in the corresponding Element. It is important to have a balance of flavours in our diet so that no one flavour is either absent or dominant.

Colour
Yellow

In China, where the Five Element system originated, the colour yellow was associated with the colour of soil, ploughed earth and the famous Yellow River. This waterway is famous for silting up, its high soil content producing the yellow colour. The golden-brownish yellow of a field of ripening grain is emblematic of both the colour and ripe fullness of the Earth Element.

In clothing, yellow is less common and yellow garments are rarely fashionable in Western countries. Perhaps this colour does not suit people with pale skin. Yellow clothing is more common in Asian and African countries where the bright colour goes well with darker skin tones.

What is your feeling about yellow? Do you have any yellow in your wardrobe? When might you choose to wear yellow clothes? How much yellow is in your home? It is good to have some yellow in your surroundings. According to *feng shui* principles, while the other four Elements relate to the four walls of a room, the Earth Element rules the middle of the room. Some yellow cushions, yellow-flowers on a table or some yellow in a tablecloth can bring Earth energy into a room. The kitchen is more closely related to Earth since it is the place where nourishing food is prepared. Bringing yellow-coloured and earth-toned objects into the kitchen is very beneficial to the energy of the home.

In Five Element diagnosis, a yellow colour in the face can indicate an imbalance in the Spleen and Stomach, the organs of Earth. The presence of dampness in the Spleen can often be observed as yellow around the mouth or cheeks.[5] People of an Earth constitution will exhibit a yellow colour at the sides of the eyes. This colour can range from the bright yellow of a canary to a muddy, brown colour and sometimes appears as the colour of cream where the yellow is almost white.

Sound
Singing

The sound of the Earth voice is one that has the widest variation. While the Wood and Fire voices are predominantly up and the Metal and Water voices are predominantly down, the Earth voice goes both up and down, often in the same sentence.

The sound of someone's voice is diagnostic of their Constitutional Element and those of an Earth constitution will reveal this singing voice. The sound of singing carries the emotion of sympathy. Imagine a mother expressing sympathy to her child who has just fallen over. Such a tone would be caring, soothing, rounded in shape, not harsh. Think also of a rider soothing a frightened horse and how that voice would be modulated and soft.

People of an Earth constitution will demonstrate this singing quality in their normal speaking voice. Even if they are talking about something sad or something that made them angry or afraid, the sing-song quality will show through.

There are some cultures in which people naturally speak in this way. The Welsh accent is a prime example of the singing voice. Scandinavians who speak English often sound as if their voice is going up and down in rapid alternation. In such cases, we must compare the person's voice to the norm within their culture. Not all people from Wales are Earth types!

Odour
Fragrant

A person's subtle body odour is the third of the diagnostic tools that help to identify a person's Constitutional Element. Those of an Earth constitution will emanate an odour that is described as fragrant, though this description is quite misleading. It is not the smell of fresh-cut roses or honeysuckle in spring. While a healthy Earth person will have an odour that is somewhat sweet, it tends towards an excessive sweetness that can be cloying or sickly. When the person is out of balance, the odour becomes even stronger and can resemble that of fermenting grain or even baby's vomit.

The odour arises from the organs of the Constitutional Element not doing their job optimally. In this case, it is the Stomach that is not functioning well enough to digest properly, producing an odour of partially digested food.

Emotion
Sympathy
and worry

Traditional Chinese medicine regards worry as the emotion of Earth. Sometimes it is described as pensiveness or over-thinking. Like the planet Earth, the activity of worry goes round and round in ceaseless repetition. This overactive mental activity injures the Spleen.[6] It also keeps too much energy in the head, leaving the worrier top-heavy and ungrounded, out of contact with the belly, legs and feet.

In the Five Element tradition, the emotion assigned to Earth is sympathy. This divergence occurred in the 1960s when acupuncture was first practised in England. The only English translation of the *Neijing* available at that time was Ilza Veith's 1949 edition which substitutes sympathy for worry.[7] This was perpetuated by Felix Mann's 1963 book on acupuncture,[8] which in turn influenced J.R. Worsley's understanding.[9]

In following this translation of the character as sympathy, Worsley discovered that people of an Earth constitution tend to be out of balance in this emotion. At one extreme they can be overly sympathetic towards other people. They focus on the needs of others at the expense of their own needs and in ways that are more concerned with their own need to give than the other's need to receive. At the other extreme, the Earth person can be characteristically unsympathetic to the needs and sufferings of other people, becoming self-focused, selfish and narcissistic.

Some argue that worry is not really an emotion at all but rather a mental activity. Worry does not produce the intense movements of Qi as do the emotions of fear, anger, joy and grief, and therefore sympathy more accurately describes the core emotion of Earth.[10] Nonetheless, worry has a profound impact on the Earth energies and cannot be ignored.

Organs and officials

The Earth organs of Stomach and Spleen have a central place because together they form an axis in the body. The Stomach is the most important of the yang organs.[11] It is referred to as the Great Granary and is responsible for the nourishment of all the other organs.[12] This gives it much more importance in Chinese medicine.

To begin with, it controls receiving. This includes the taking in of food and holding on to it, but it also extends to receiving things such as love, support and appreciation. Second, Stomach begins the process of transformation of food into food essence which Spleen will transport throughout the body. Third, Stomach controls the descent of Qi, ensuring the proper downward movement of food and the movement of Qi down the body.

The yin organ of Earth is Spleen which assists the Stomach in transforming food into energy and moving this around the body. It is also charged with moving Qi and fluids. Therefore, the Spleen official can be regarded as the Minister for Transport.

The second function of the Spleen is to control ascending Qi which supports an upright lift to the body. When Spleen Qi is weak, fatigue is often a result. The state of the Spleen is one of the most important factors in determining the amount of energy a person has.[13]

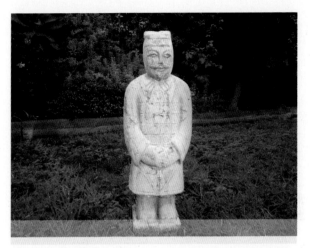

*An army marches
on its Stomach 36*

One of the most potent acupoints of all lies on the
Stomach meridian. Its Chinese name *Zusanli* is
translated as Leg Three Miles. It was a point
reputedly used by ancient Chinese soldiers to
enable them to go the extra three miles in their
marches. For not only does this point power the
legs, but by drawing on reserves of strength it
fortifies the whole body, tonifying the Qi and
eliminating fatigue.

Zusanli
LEG THREE
MILES
Stomach 36

What is more, *Zusanli* treats most digestive
conditions including nausea, vomiting, reflux,
belching, stomach cramps, bloating, flatulence,
diarrhoea, low appetite and poor digestion. If that's
not enough, it improves the immune system and
treats chills, fever and asthma.

This is such a powerful point that it is said
that by the daily stimulation of this point you can
live to be 100. (Let me know if it works for you!)
Qin Cheng-zu, a physician in the 5th century CE,
claimed that by using ST 36 all diseases can be

treated.[14] It is a veritable Swiss army knife, with many tools rolled into one.

Modern studies of the use of acupuncture on ST 36 have demonstrated that stimulation of the point produces measurable changes in the areas of the brain related to gastric function.[15]

As the Earth point of an Earth meridian, ST 36 balances the Element and allows greater access to the qualities of the Earth. Thus, it gives a greater sense of solidity, stability and grounding, both physically and emotionally. It supports a person's capacity to receive nourishment, both from food and from other people. It balances the mania and depression of bipolar disorder, and calms agitation and other emotions such as anger, fright and sadness.

Zusanli has a substantial influence on the pathway of the Stomach meridian and so can treat conditions as diverse as tension in the jaw, abscess and swelling in the breast, issues of the abdomen and pain in the thigh, knee and lower leg.

One of my clients was an amateur soccer player who would come for treatment two days before a big game. He always reminded me to 'do the three miles point' for he found it helped him to run further on the field and to recover more quickly after the game. His experience was a modern equivalent of those ancient soldiers who were able to march further by supporting the Stomach meridian.

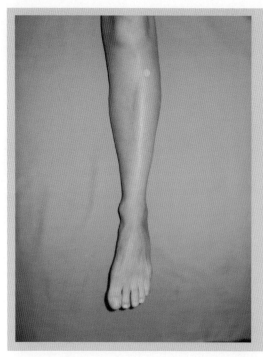

Location of
Stomach 36

The point is 3 cun below the base of the patella and
a finger's width lateral to the crest of the tibia. With
the leg straight, place the side of your index finger
at the base of the kneecap. Where the edge of your
little finger comes to rest, go to the outside of the
ridge of the leg bone by a finger's width. The point
is located in the tibialis anterior (shin muscle).
Use firm, direct pressure or massage in a clockwise
direction.

Combines with SP 3 · SP 4 · ST 13 ·
ST 25 · ST 40 · GB 21

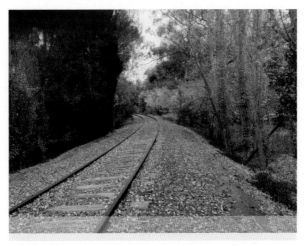

Transport yourself

Taibai
SUPREME
WHITE
Spleen 3

Years ago when industrial strike action was common, there was nothing more paralysing than a transportation strike. Planes grounded, trains halted, ports closed, trucks idle. The transport of people and goods is vital to the functioning of a country and its economy.

In the human body, the job of moving things around falls to the Spleen official. Of all the organs, the Spleen is the most unlike its Western namesake. In fact, it can be regarded more like a network than an organ such as the liver. Think of a subway map with its network of criss-crossing lines. Spleen is like the Minister for Transport who keeps things moving.

The main function of the Spleen is to assist the Stomach in the transformation of food essences and to transport these throughout the body. It is also responsible for the movements of Qi and fluids. When the Spleen Qi is strong, there will be good appetite, digestion and elimination. When it is weak, there may be poor digestion, bloating and loose stools.

Another function of the Spleen is to control ascending Qi, partnering the Stomach's role of controlling descending Qi. One way this operates is that the Spleen sends food Qi upwards to the Lung to support its function of gathering Qi from the breath. It also sends food Qi upwards to the Heart to assist in forming Blood. In an overall way, the Spleen provides support and upward lift to the body.

One interpretation of the pathway of the Spleen meridian is that it is like a crutch under the armpit, supporting an upright stance. When Spleen Qi is weak, there is often fatigue and sagging as if this upright support has been lost.

When the functions of transformation, transportation and ascendance of Qi are operating well, then thinking is clear and the thoughts are settled. When the Spleen official is taking a sick day, then the mind can become fuzzy and muddled, worried by repetitive and obsessive thoughts.

Disorders of the Spleen are common and Spleen Qi deficiency is one of the most common patterns seen in clinical acupuncture practice in Western countries. Causes of this include stress, lack of exercise, poor diet, eating too much sugar, eating cold food, eating irregularly and worrying about what you eat. Looking at this list, it is easy to see how this has become a Western malaise.

One of the strongest points for tonifying and revitalising the Spleen is its source point, *Taibai* – Supreme White. As the Earth point on an Earth meridian, it is tremendously supportive of the Element and particularly effective between the hours of 9am and 11am when the Spleen Qi is at its highest level during the day.

It activates and strengthens the Qi of both Spleen and Stomach, thereby treating many digestive disorders including abdominal pain and fullness, intestinal gurgling (borborygmus), constipation, diarrhoea and haemorrhoids. By encouraging the Qi to ascend, *Taibai* also treats lethargy, fatigue and feelings of heaviness in the body, especially of the limbs. It also treats pain of the knees and thighs along the pathways of Stomach and Spleen.

Taibai is a good point for resolving damp. The Spleen is particularly susceptible to external damp, such as humid weather or wearing wet clothes. But internal damp often arises when the Spleen is not functioning well. Many of the symptoms of Spleen imbalance are a result of this dampness in the body.

The Spleen is also injured by ongoing obsessive thoughts and excessive worry. In these cases, *Taibai* helps to recharge the brain and the thinking processes. It brightens up your ideas! Similarly, when thinking is fuzzy and mental activity is fraught, this point clarifies thinking and improves memory. It brings grounding, stability and a sense of coming back to centre.

If you feel as if your inner transport minister has gone on strike, hold *Taibai* and get him back to work.

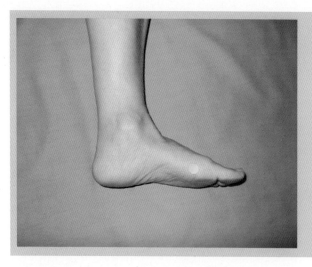

Location of
Spleen 3

The point is located on the inside of the foot below
the ball of the big toe. It lies on the side of the foot
at the junction of the red and white skin. Press into
the depression at the base of the big toe.

Combines with ST 36 · ST 40 · SP 4 ·
SP 6 · SP 21 · BL 49

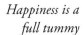

Happiness is a full tummy

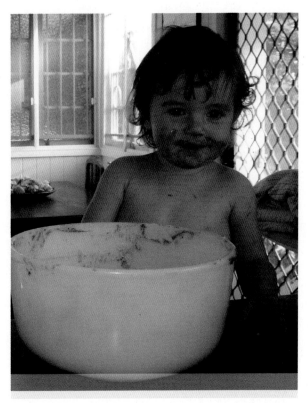

Fenglong
ABUNDANT
SPLENDOUR

Stomach 40

Imagine that you have just eaten a delicious meal of fresh food, cooked and seasoned to perfection, a perfect balance of flavours and textures. As you push away from the table, you feel completely sated, humming with contentment. This sense of satisfaction from an abundance of nourishment is one of the qualities to be found in a balanced Earth Element. It applies not only to food, but to being satisfied in all areas of life.

The Chinese character for stomach is *wei,* depicting a stomach with food inside it, suggesting that a full tummy is the natural state of things. It echoes the description in the *Nan-ching* of the Stomach as the Great Granary.[16]

The Earth organs of Stomach and Spleen hold a special importance because together they form a central axis in the body. The Stomach is the most important of the yang organs and is responsible for the nourishment of all the other organs. The *Neijing* says that the five yin organs and six yang organs derive their Qi and nutrition from the Stomach.[17] The Stomach therefore has a wider significance and influence in Chinese medicine than from the Western perspective.

For example, it controls receiving. This function goes beyond merely being a repository for food taken in through the mouth. The Stomach is responsible for appetite which prompts the desire to take in food and also holds on to the food once it is ingested. Weak Stomach receiving may produce poor appetite, reflux and belching. This function of receiving also extends to the emotional level and the capacity to receive support and love from others.

The Stomach controls the rotting and ripening of food and drink, a process of transformation. Then the Stomach, together with the Spleen, controls the transport of the essences of food throughout the body. To have strong Stomach Qi is synonymous with robust health, while weak Stomach Qi will produce fatigue and ill health.

The Stomach also controls the descent of Qi. If the Qi does not properly descend, food will stagnate and produce bloating and belching. The Stomach is responsible not only for the downward movement of food to the Small Intestine, but also more generally for the movement of Qi down the body. When the Stomach is not performing this task, there is a counter-flow of Qi which ascends rather than descends.

An acupoint that serves to balance the Stomach official as well as the organ is *Fenglong* – Abundant Splendour. As the *luo*-connecting point of Stomach meridian, *Fenglong* connects to its partner Spleen and balances Qi between the two, harmonising the yin and yang of Earth.

It is the single most important point for clearing phlegm from the body. Phlegm arises when the Spleen's function of transportation of fluids is impaired and fluid congeals. As the connecting point, *Fenglong* activates the Spleen's transporting function and so treats phlegm-related conditions, particularly of the digestive and respiratory systems: cough with mucous, bronchitis, pneumonia, constipation, nausea, vomiting, gastric pain, cysts, lipomas and other lumps under the skin.

But it is for its effects in the psycho-emotional realm that *Fenglong* is renowned in the Five Element tradition. It helps a person who is feeling scarcity in her life to reconnect with a sense of abundance. The character *feng* depicts the threshing floor at harvest time, brimming with grain, while *long* indicates a multiplication manyfold of this abundance.[18] Together they portray the magnificent, splendorous bounty of heaven and earth.

Ultimately, the feeling of abundance has nothing to do with how much we possess, for abundance is not a physical state, but a condition of the mind and of the spirit. When Earth energies are balanced, there is a natural recognition of the abundance that the universe offers us: the bounty and the beauty of nature, the love and connection we share with others, and the simple fact of being alive. Abundant Splendour proclaims these gifts of Earth. It has the capacity to connect us with the truth that we *are* already the cornucopia of life's abundance. When we understand that we are a living personification of abundance, there can be deep satisfaction from simply being alive and present to life.

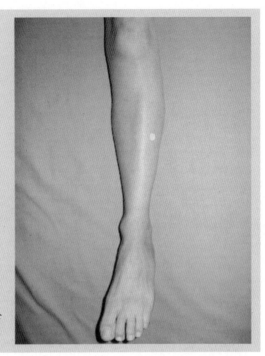

Location of
Stomach 40

The point is on the outside of the leg, halfway
between the knee crease and the ankle bone and
two fingers' width lateral to the crest of the tibia
bone. Use firm, direct pressure.

Combines with ST 13 · ST 25 ·
ST 36 · SP 3 · SP 4

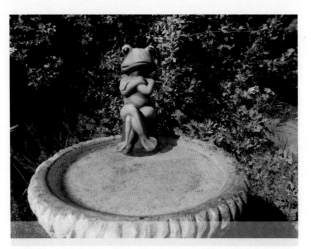

Master of the seas

In our demanding, fast-paced, modern world, stress can produce tension in the organs and tissues of the abdomen, affecting digestion and elimination as well as the reproductive organs.

Gongsun
GRANDFATHER
GRANDSON
Spleen 4

In *Gongsun* – Grandfather Grandson, we find a point that acts upon the abdomen in multiple ways. It is a powerful point of the Spleen channel and the *luo*-connecting point of that meridian. And it is the master point of the *Chong Mai* (Penetrating Vessel) which influences the whole of the abdomen and all its organs.

Its name alone alerts us to its prominence in the pantheon of points. *Gongsun* was the family name of the legendary Yellow Emperor Huang Di, whose conversations with his physicians form the basis of the *Neijing*, that towering classic of Taoism and Chinese medicine. The translation of Grandfather Grandson suggests continuity through the generations. At a mundane level it uses the analogy of the grandson for the connecting channel, which is an offshoot of its grandfather, the Spleen channel.[19]

Yellow is the colour of Earth and the Yellow Emperor was said to have ruled during the Earth phase of China's history. His reign laid the foundations for Chinese civilisation in the same way that the Earth Element is the base and orientation of all the other Elements.

Whichever explanation of the name we wish to take, *Gongsun* is a potent point for influencing the Earth Element and its organs of Stomach and Spleen. It is particularly effective in combination with ST 40, the *luo*-connecting point of Stomach meridian. By activating the Spleen, it treats lethargy, fatigue, chronic tiredness and weakness.

Like other connecting points of the yin meridians, SP 4 exerts a pronounced influence over the emotions.[20] Because of Spleen's connection to the Heart, SP 4 can settle the spirit when there is restlessness, agitation, insomnia, mania and depression. The point also addresses an imbalance of sympathy, where a person suffers self-pity and feels unsupported by others and by the world at large, or relies too heavily on others to meet their needs.

Already we can see that *Gongsun* is an influential point. But there is more. Another of its roles is as master point of the *Chong Mai* (Penetrating Vessel), one of the Eight Extraordinary Vessels.

The Vessels are fields of Qi as opposed to the rivers of Qi that are the meridians. *Gongsun* exerts an influence over the entire field of the Penetrating Vessel which extends throughout the torso from the pubis to the throat and includes the spinal column and the insides of the legs. The Penetrating Vessel is described as both the sea of Blood and the sea of the meridians. It therefore exerts a strong regulating effect on Blood and Qi.[21]

As the master point of the sea of Blood, SP 4 regulates blood circulation, stops bleeding and addresses all menstrual irregularities. It has an influence on the uterus and treats gynaecological disorders such as endometriosis, fibroids and cysts.

As the master point of the sea of the meridians, it ensures good circulation of Qi throughout the twelve meridians. It addresses counter-flow Qi – for example, where Stomach Qi is rising rather than descending and causing chest or gastric pain.

It is believed that the Extraordinary Vessels develop at conception and form the basis of the energy network of the body, well before the development of the twelve organ meridians.[22] Treating the Vessels therefore treats the depth and foundation of who we are as humans.

Spend some time with *Gongsun* and become master of your own inner seas.

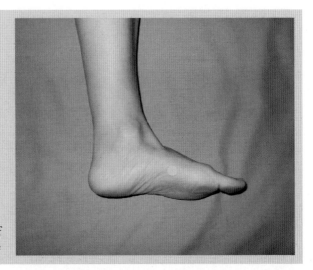

Location of
Spleen 4

In the arch of the foot, in a depression at the base of the first metatarsal bone. Find Spleen 3 in a depression at the ball of the toe, then slide your finger up the shaft of the metatarsal until you are at the base of the bone. Apply firm pressure directed towards the ankle.

Combines with ST 36 · ST 40 · SP 3 · SP 6 · SP 21 · HP 6

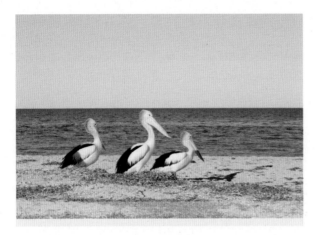

*One for all,
all for one*

The motto of the Three Musketeers could well be applied to *Sanyinjiao* – Three Yin Crossing, where three meridians unite at a single point. While the point is given to the Spleen meridian because its primary influence is upon the Spleen, it is a meeting point with the Kidney and Liver meridians. Like a river that joins together with two other tributaries, producing a combined force, SP 6 is a powerful confluence of forces where the combined action is more than the sum of the parts.

Sanyinjiao
THREE YIN
CROSSING
Spleen 6

** Forbidden during
pregnancy*

The wide range of conditions addressed by this point makes it one of the most frequently selected points in treatment. As it influences the three yin meridians of the leg, it treats conditions of the digestive, urinary, lymphatic and reproductive systems, treats damp, tonifies Qi and Blood, and raises the Qi upwards.

As a Spleen point, it strengthens the Spleen, thereby treating all symptoms of Spleen Qi deficiency: feelings of heaviness and fatigue, abdominal fullness, loss of appetite and loose bowels. It clears oedema by mobilising the Spleen's capacity to move fluids. Similarly, it has a strong influence on nourishing the Blood and clearing Blood stagnation.

Three Yin Crossing is a great point for resolving damp, a pathogenic factor to which the Spleen is particularly prone. Damp in the lower burner can manifest as infections of the bladder, vagina and prostate; damp in the middle burner can cause diarrhoea, poor digestion, abdominal pain and nausea.

In its role as a Kidney point, it strengthens Kidney Qi which is the source of our vitality. It treats difficult and painful urination, tinnitus, night sweats, dry mouth and difficulty with hot weather.

As a Liver point, it promotes the smooth flow of Liver Qi, treats painful menstruation and abdominal pain generally. It also treats pain in the genitals, seminal emission and sexual hyperactivity in men, impotence and infertility, blurred vision and hypertension.

Sanyinjiao is one of the best points for regulating the uterus, and so is very useful for all menstrual irregularities. Its effect on the uterus makes it one of the best points for promoting labour, and is therefore forbidden during pregnancy except in the final stages.

Emotionally, it soothes the spirit when a person is despairing, feeling weighed down by the burdens of life. It helps calm a worried mind and ease insomnia. Its influence over the Liver means it can calm irritability, especially when associated with premenstrual syndrome (PMS).

Spleen 6 combines well with Stomach 36 to strengthen the middle burner and balance the Earth Element. A nice little treatment is to combine Spleen 6 with the source points of the three associated meridians, namely Spleen 3, Kidney 3 and Liver 3. The quality of the Qi at these three points will tell you much about the health of these meridians and organs.

If you want to raise your game, raise your Qi with this Triple Crown winner of a point.

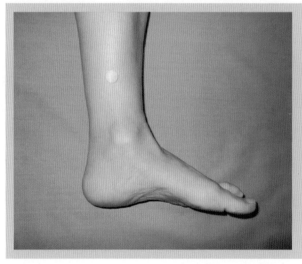

Location of
Spleen 6

Located 3 cun (four fingers' width) above the crest of the inner ankle bone. Press towards the back of the tibia bone.

Combines with SP 3 · LV 3 · K 3 · ST 36

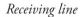

Receiving line

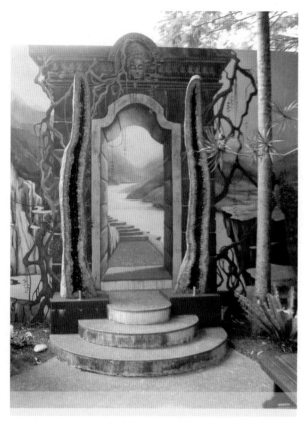

Qihu
QI DOOR
Stomach 13

There is a tradition at weddings known as the receiving line, when guests line up to offer the newlywed couple their congratulations and wishes. The couple in turn thank them for their attendance and gifts.

The upper reaches of the Stomach channel are a kind of receiving line in the body, where the Qi passes through the cheeks, jaw and throat before going through the Qi Door and moving down through the chest and abdomen. The gifts received are the Qi from food and the breath.

The Stomach channel makes its way on to the chest at *Qihu* – Qi Door. When this point is blocked, Qi can become congested in the upper points of the Stomach channel, those in the cheeks, jaw, temples and throat. Opening this door can allow the Qi to flow freely down the meridian, through the chest, abdomen and legs to the feet.

For people who are great givers but who have difficulty receiving from others, this point can support receiving at many levels. To begin with, it helps if there is difficulty swallowing, enhancing the ability to take in food. By opening the upper chest, it allows a person to breathe more deeply and therefore receive more of the Heavenly Qi that comes with the breath. At the psychological level, *Qihu* supports a person to receive sympathy, compliments and love, and to take in all that life has to give.

For people of an Earth constitution and for those whose Earth Element is shaky, there can be difficulty finding a balance between giving and receiving. Most often this appears as a tendency to over-give to others at the expense of themselves – giving too much, giving inappropriately, giving when it is not wanted. At the same time they are unable to receive easily from others. This might appear as discomfort in accepting help, denying there is any help needed, or feeling compelled to give something of equal or greater value in return.

In these cases, *Qihu* can support the person to receive more easily. Healthy receiving is that which has gratitude for the gift and is open and gracious. It receives without a feeling of entitlement to that which is given or a sense of guilt at receiving the gift. And it does not react by feeling a need to give something back in return.

At the physical level, this point helps to relax the neck and throat. I use this point quite frequently as part of the five-step neck release. When held with a slight downward pressure, it enables a subtle release of the fascia at the front of the neck and of the scalene muscles. This in turn can take pressure off the back of the neck where there is stiffness and difficulty turning the head.

It also treats fullness of the chest and ribcage, pain in the chest and upper back, and respiratory conditions such as cough, asthma, wheezing and bronchitis.

Find out what's behind your Qi Door!

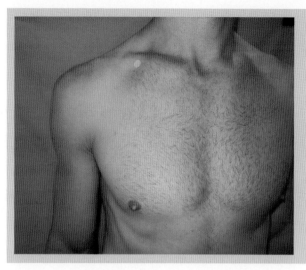

Location of
Stomach 13

The point lies directly below the clavicle, 4 cun
lateral to the midline and in line with the nipple.
Apply direct pressure or angle slightly downward.

Combines with ST 25 · ST 36 · ST 40 ·
any point in the back or side of the neck

*And fill all fruit
with ripeness
to the core*

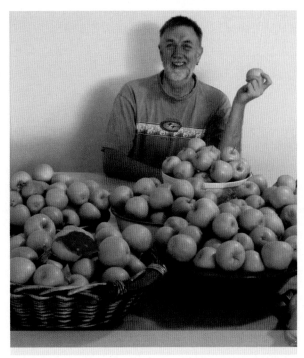

When Keats penned his 'Ode to Autumn',[23] much of his poem evoked the rich, full ripeness of harvest time. He wrote of mellow fruitfulness, swelling gourds, plumped hazelnuts, vines loaded with fruit, and a profusion of flowers for the bees. All of these images are richly redolent of the Earth Element.

The season of Earth is that of the late summer or harvest time, when the year-long efforts of farmers and gardeners are rewarded with the bounty of the fruits of the earth. This harvest of the Earth Element is dependent on the full flourishing of the summer Fire, which in turn is dependent on the rapid springtime growth of Wood. This in turn is founded on the restoration and rejuvenation of the Water in winter.

But sometimes, despite all efforts, harvests fail, resulting in pain and sorrow, lack of sustenance and nurturance. This is true not only in the planting of crops, but of life more generally. Sometimes our best-laid plans come to nothing.

J.R. Worsley observed that many people of an Earth constitution have a pervasive sense that their plans, hopes and dreams seldom produce a satisfying outcome or feeling of fulfilment. It is as if the whole span of life is in some way deeply unsatisfying. Worsley coined the term 'lack of harvest' to describe this feature, and it has become diagnostic of an Earth constitution.

Imagine yourself as a farmer who sows crops, tends them with care for months, only to see the plants ruined by drought, floods, pests or disease. All that love and labour come to nothing. Imagine the sorrow that the farmer feels at the loss.

Now imagine that same sorrow repeated over and over again until it seems that one's whole life is a failed harvest.

For the person whose life appears this way, *Fuai* – Abdomen Sorrow – can be a powerful point. It addresses the beliefs that needs will never be satisfied, and that life is a barren field where nothing ever grows to maturity. Where this is the case, this point can provide support and nurturance for the Earth Element, not just in the Earth type but in all of us.

At the physical level, *Fuai* is traditionally used to treat an unhappy tummy, plagued with the pain of indigestion and bloating. One translation of the name, Abdominal Lament, suggests an abdomen crying out in pain. Indeed, sometimes obstructions in the intestines do produce a sound like weeping.

At a spiritual level, the point can become a portal to the understanding that our needs are only fully satisfied when we connect with the depth of our true self. From this depth, we need nothing. To live from our true nature is complete and total fulfilment.

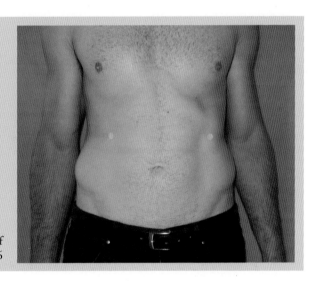

Location of
Spleen 16

Located on the abdomen, on the nipple line, 4 cun lateral to and 3 cun above the navel. The point lies on the edge of the rectus abdominus muscle. Use gentle, direct pressure.

Combines with SP 3 · SP 4 · SP 21 · ST 40

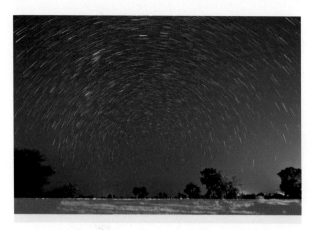

Tianshu is the name the Chinese gave to the star Dubhe, which forms part of the Big Dipper or Plough in the northern night sky. This star is used as a pointer to Polaris, the North Star, around which the heavens appear to pivot.

Tianshu
HEAVENLY
PIVOT
Stomach 25

This notion of pivoting around a centre is apt for the acupoint *Tianshu* – Heavenly Pivot, which lies at the level of the navel. The point points to the umbilicus, our energetic centre, the original connection to our mother who was the earthly source and centre of our world in childhood.

This characteristic of centrality is, well, central to the nature of the Earth Element. We see this expressed at all levels of its manifestation. At the physical level, the organs of Stomach and Spleen are central to digestion and lie in the middle of the body. Emotionally, Earth wants to mediate and to connect others together. At a cosmic level, it provides the pivotal point of balance between the heavens and the mundane world.

Physically, *Tianshu* is a highly effective point for stomach and intestinal problems. Deadman goes so far as to call it the single most important point for the treatment of the widest variety of intestinal disorders.[24]

As the front-*mu* point of the Large Intestine, it treats conditions such as constipation and diarrhoea. At this meeting point, the functions of Stomach and Large Intestine intersect, harmonising the processes of digestion and elimination.

Tianshu also treats endometriosis, abdominal masses and menstrual disorders. And it ameliorates the lethargy and fatigue of Spleen Qi deficiency.

As the celestial pivot, it balances the yang of the upper body with the yin of the lower body. For those who are energetically top-heavy, ungrounded and relatively absent from their legs and feet, this is a great grounding point. When there is a lot of repetitive, obsessive thought, this point helps to draw the focus away from the head. For those who are energetically bottom-heavy, the point helps to raise the Spleen Qi, supporting vitality and activity.

Tianshu is a good point for emotional volatility and where there are big swings in mood and energy levels. It treats a condition known in Chinese medicine as 'running piglet Qi' where there is a sensation of agitation and tightness in the abdomen as if tiny piglets were running madly between navel and the throat. This condition is exacerbated by stress, sexual repression and unexpressed emotion. Therefore, the point is used in psychosomatic problems when there is abdominal distress.[25] Running piglet Qi is often a diagnosis for panic attack.

A characteristic of the Earth Element is that it facilitates transitions and this point is especially helpful in supporting someone who is going through a life transition by helping to keep them stable and centred with a grounded connection to the earth.

When you feel that you have become ungrounded or uncentred, or have left yourself in some way, you can return to centre by focusing on this point of pivot which balances the celestial Qi with the earthly Qi. Become balanced between heaven and earth.

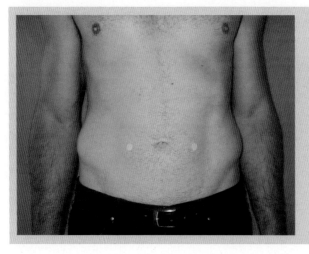

Location of
Stomach 25

The point is located at the level of the navel and 2 cun lateral to it. It is halfway from the navel to the border of the rectus abdominus muscle. Apply moderate, direct pressure.

Combines with ST 13 · ST 36 ·
ST 40 · SP 3 · BL 25 · LI 4

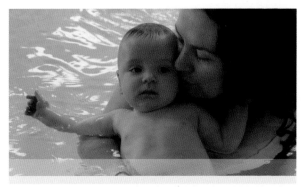

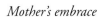
Mother's embrace

Dabao
GREAT
ENVELOPING
Spleen 21

Hugs come in many forms: a light greeting, a supportive holding, an affectionate embrace, a passionate clinch, a mother's love-you-to-bits squeeze. A loving, caring, full-frontal hug sees the arms enfold the other person, wrapping around the back and sides, while the two chests meet. What is common to all these hugs is caring. You enfold the other person in your arms in a caring embrace. You care for their wellbeing. Such caring is the essence of the Earth Element.

The Earth qualities of caring, support and nourishment are amply demonstrated and demonstrably amplified at the acupoint *Dabao* – Great Enveloping, which lies on the side of the ribcage. Imagine a mother embracing her child, arms wrapped around the little body, holding and squeezing with maternal love. The child's entire upper body is enveloped, wrapped in mother's love.

The character of *Dabao* includes a pictogram of a foetus in the womb to suggest something contained within, wrapped up or enveloped. A foetus receives holding, support and nourishment, all essential qualities of Earth.

Dabao transmits these essences by virtue of its role as the point of the Great Spleen Connecting Channel. This channel arises at SP 21 and radiates throughout the chest, through what are known as the minute collaterals, enveloping the chest with Qi and Blood, and supporting the Heart. The point relieves fullness, oppression and depression in the Heart area, bringing a feeling of freedom, openness, harmony and togetherness. It effects an internal, enfolding, motherly embrace.

This function of moving Qi and Blood extends throughout the body because Dabao controls all the *luo*-connecting points. We have looked at a number of *luo*-connecting points so far and seen how these points balance the yin and yang of their Element. In SP 21 we have the Great-*luo* point, the mother of all connecting points. In this role, it treats the whole network of connecting channels and their Blood, thereby nourishing the whole body. In this way, it treats muscular pain that moves throughout the body as well as looseness of the joints.[26]

Another major function of *Dabao* is as the exit point of the Spleen meridian. From here, the Qi moves into the entry point of Heart meridian at Heart 1 – Utmost Source, which lies in the centre of the armpit. Here is another way that Spleen nourishes the Heart, through the *wei-qi* cycle.

Spleen 21 needs to be open in order to serve the Heart, and Heart 1 needs to be open to receive the nourishment.

When Qi becomes blocked at points of exit or entry, an entry/exit block occurs and poses a significant impediment to effective treatment. The Spleen/Heart block is one of the most common of these blocks. Symptoms of such a block can include fullness of the chest, palpitations, pain in the ribcage, pain in the armpit, skin eruptions at or between the points, appetite disorders, fatigue and depression.

Something I have discovered through bodywork is that by holding both SP 21 points simultaneously, a gentle myofascial compression is created. When this hold is maintained for about three minutes, the fascia of the whole ribcage begins to unwind, contributing greatly to the effect that SP 21 has on freeing the Qi of the chest.

This can be done by using gentle pressure with the palms over the points, a hold which often feels very comforting to the recipient, like a supportive, caring embrace.

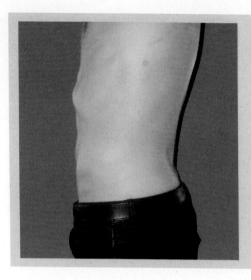

Location of
Spleen 21

On the very side of the ribcage, below the armpit, in the seventh intercostal space (some sources locate in the sixth intercostal space). It lies roughly at the level of the xiphoid process at the base of the sternum. The point can be held with moderate, direct pressure or with the palm as suggested above.

Combines with SP 3 · SP 4 · H 7

The spirit of Earth

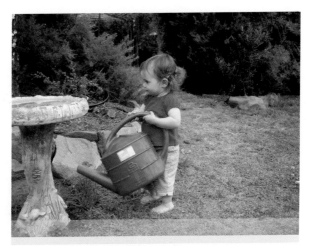

Yi, the spirit of Earth, is most often translated as intention, thought or intellect. It is the spirit which supports the manifestation of new things to come into being. It unifies thought and action into a form of doing that, with applied purpose, produces desired ends.

The character *yi* has two parts. The upper part depicts an uttered sound, such as a word or a musical note. The lower part depicts the heart. The character therefore portrays the intention of a man who speaks, manifested by the sounds he utters.[27] This intention emanates from the heart, suggesting that the spoken words are founded on the sincerity and integrity of the speaker.

The *Neijing* says that the Spleen houses the *yi*,[28] and therefore anything that injures the Spleen will also injure the *yi*. Incessant worry is most injurious and undermines the steadiness of a balanced Earth.

Going round and round in the head or chewing over something repeatedly will erode the *yi*. The resulting imbalance can cause a person to feel confusion, lethargy, boredom or indifference. Alternatively, it can manifest as exaggerated sympathy, stickiness in relationships and uncontrolled or even self-destructive generosity.[29]

One of the important qualities of intention is steadiness. The continued, sustained application of intention towards a goal is needed for the desired outcome to be achieved. It is the glue that sticks the writer to his chair in order to complete the manuscript; it is what gets the athlete to training day in and day out; and it is what supports a mother to keep on being there for her children as she rears them to adulthood. It is the *yi* which sustains a practice of any kind, whether it is playing the violin, working on your backhand or sitting on the meditation cushion each morning. It provides us with the support to keep on keeping on with the things we commit ourselves to.

The Earth qualities of intention, steadiness and application are particularly evoked by the outer *shu* point of the Spleen, *Yishe* – Thought Dwelling. This point influences the *yi*, translated here as thought, but encompassing the quality of intention described earlier. Kaptchuck calls *yi* the consciousness of potentials, the highest form of thought 'that is responsible for considering, deliberating and deciding on what is likely, possible or conceivable'.[30]

The left-hand character *yi* contains the heart radical at the bottom. It can be translated as meaning 'the process of establishing meaning in the world with words that come from the heart'.[31] *Yi* is not simply about thinking but includes the bringing of thought into manifestation through the vehicle of intention.

When these qualities of a healthy Earth Element become constrained and obscured by worry, repetitive thoughts and obsessions; when the mind is stuck in a rut and cannot get out of it; if there is stubbornness; if the mind is foggy, hazy and leaden, unable to process thoughts effectively; or if the person has lost their centre, swayed this way and that by all around them, then *Yishe* will help. It supports the Spleen to understand, grasp and work sequentially along a passage of thought. It helps us to digest our life experience in a way that is meaningful and will support fruitful action in the world. And it supports steadiness of intention that manifests a person's purpose.

At a physical level, *Yishe* supports the digestive system. It treats abdominal fullness and distension, diarrhoea, gastroenteritis, difficult ingestion and vomiting.

Use this point to restore clarity of thought, sustain focused intention and support steadiness of purpose. Nourish the depths of your Earth with *Yishe*.

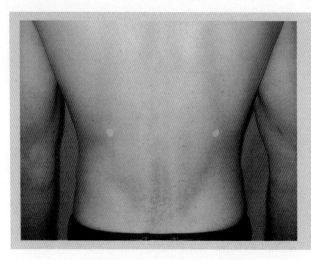

Location of
Bladder 49

Located on the back in the lower ribs and 3 cun lateral to the spine. It is level with the space between the 11th and 12th thoracic vertebrae. Use firm, direct pressure. If working on yourself, lie on a tennis ball pressing into the point.

Combines with SP 3 · SP 4 · BL 57 · BL 60

The late summer, sometimes referred to as the Indian summer, is a period of comforting warmth when the season seems to hang in the air for a time. The bees, thinking warm days will never cease, busily gather the last of the pollens as if the summer will go on forever. Nature is infused with sweet warmth, roundness and plumpness. There is a feeling of lazy languor about the days where the sun's warmth is comforting without being scorching.

Eventually, there comes a day when the comfortable warmth vanishes and there are harbingers of the change to come. There is a crispness to the days, a nip in the air and a chill to the wind. In temperate areas, the first frost arrives to snap us out of our late-summer haze. Leaves begin to leave their trees.

This transition from Earth to Metal marks the beginning of the yin half of the year's cycle, where nature's energy begins to descend and contract. Temperatures fall, leaves drop, days shorten. For many people this is the most challenging of the transitions. The falling energy of the year is a reminder that what goes up must come down. And the yin is sadly unappreciated in Western countries. Decline and decay are anathema to a culture which prizes only growth and fruition.

But for those who can appreciate and value the yin aspects of their nature – and this is fully half of who we are – this transition can seem like a welcome relief. The movement to autumn provides more space, more time to breathe. It invites reflection and contemplation, supports meditation.

The leaves that are falling from the trees outside your window inspire you to settle down.
Into yourself.

5 Metal

金

The movement of Metal is downwards.

After the uprising yang of Wood and Fire and the balanced axis of Earth, Metal represents the beginning of yin in the *sheng* cycle. Metal is representative of precious metals such as gold and silver, precious gems, crystals and minerals, all of which are stored underground, treasures awaiting discovery.

In the human body, Metal manifests as the minerals and trace minerals that are essential for biochemistry and the maintenance of health and life. We need minerals such as calcium, magnesium, copper, zinc, chromium and molybdenum. These minerals become available to us through plant and animal food sources, but all of them originate in the soil, hidden in the earth.

Metals can be fashioned into tools and weapons. The quintessential metal tool is the knife which is used for cutting away what is not needed from that which is required: peeling vegetables, scaling fish, cutting slices of pie, whittling wood. We even talk about budget cuts, tax cuts and spending cuts. Surgeons use the scalpel to cut away diseased tissue. All of these operations imply reduction, decrease, a dropping away of something in order to preserve what is essential to life.

At a metaphysical level, Metal represents the hidden treasure of our true nature. There are countless tales of heroes and heroines defeating monsters and enduring terrible ordeals in search of precious treasures. The Golden Fleece, the Holy Grail, the dragon's hoard, rings of power and magical artefacts; these are all are metaphors for the priceless treasure of wisdom, self-knowledge and realisation which are obtained by cutting through the veils of ego and delusion.

The Chinese character for Metal is *jin*. It represents nuggets of gold hidden within the earth. The symbol for the Earth Element is contained within the symbol for Metal, with an additional line suggesting greater depth, and a sloping roof indicating concealment underground. Overall, the suggestion is of something of value hidden within.[1]

The characteristics of autumn evoke the qualities of Metal.

Fall. In North America autumn is referred to as fall, a word which succinctly describes the fundamental energy of Metal. In autumn everything is falling: the leaves, the temperature, the angle of the sun. Following the prolific expansion of summer and the warm fullness of harvest time, autumn begins the descent, the turning inwards. There is a sense of quieting. Autumn invites us to ponder the impermanence of all phenomena.

Decay. The leaves and fruits of the trees drop to earth and begin to decay and rot. The nutrients and minerals of this material are returned to the earth to nourish future growth. Plants and trees drop the seeds that will ensure the continued survival of their species.

Space. Trees drop their leaves, leaving only bare branches. Fields which have given up their harvest lie fallow. Space is created. Space and spaciousness are qualities of Metal, which likes plenty of room to breathe.

Light. As the angle of the sun drops closer to the horizon line, the light of the sun is gentler, no longer intense. Because of the low angle of the sun, it lights up the dust particles in the air, creating a sense of something ethereal. I call this 'cathedral light', resembling shafts of light filtering down from upper windows in high-ceilinged churches.

Cool. After the intense heat of summer, autumn heralds much cooler daytime temperatures, crisp mornings and cold nights. Sweaters and coats, hats and scarves are retrieved from the back of the

Resonances of Metal

Season

Autumn or fall

closet. This is the beginning of movement from hot to cold, from yang to yin.

When does autumn begin? Depending on your latitude and climate, you can expect autumn to begin showing itself sometime in early August in the northern hemisphere and early February in the southern hemisphere. Look for the signs of autumn within yourself: a feeling of energy beginning to descend, perhaps an urge to clean, tidy and let go of things, a desire for more space, more quietude.

Sense

Smell

The olfactory receptors in the nasal cavity detect molecules in the air that trigger a response. The information is transmitted to the limbic brain, which is one of the oldest parts of the human brain, predating the thinking brain of the frontal cortex. While we may later interpret the smells in a cognitive way, the initial response is not at the level of thought, but rather of emotion, since the limbic system is the part of the brain that deals with emotions. Smells also leave long-lasting impressions and are strongly linked to memories. We label smells as good or bad depending on the memories they trigger.

There is a certain appropriateness to the fact that smell is a resonance of the Metal Element. The ancient Taoists regarded the spirit of Metal, the *po*, as the corporeal soul. This corporeal soul is the spirit that grounds us in the body. It is the only one of the five spirits that disappears at the time of death. It is the animal soul, the instinctual part of us. Smell is vital to the survival of wild animals;

金

in humans, this sense is what connects us most directly to our animal nature.

For some people, the sense of smell becomes more acute in the autumn. It is a good time to pay attention to this sense, which is often dulled by the proliferation of artificial scents in the environment. Watch how animals use their noses to give them information. Let your dog or cat teach you about getting more in touch with your animal self.

Colour
White

The colour white has long been associated with purity. The Roman priestesses of Vesta wore white, which symbolised their purity, and the early Christian church adopted this symbolism of white as the colour of sacrifice and virtue. The association of this colour with spirituality is common, from the white of priestly garments to angels, heaven and healing white light.

While in the West people tend to wear black as a sign of mourning, in the East it is white that is used at times of grief. In China when someone is gravely ill or has died, white clothes are worn, white candles are burnt and white cloths are hung over doorways in the mourning household.

How do you feel when you wear white? Is it a colour you are particularly drawn to or is it one you tend to avoid? An extreme attitude to this colour may indicate an imbalance in your Metal. Is there much white in your home? Too much white can give a sense of coldness, but some white is good to invite the qualities of Metal into your living space. According to *feng shui* principles, it is good to have some white on the Metal wall of a room, the one on your right you as you enter.

In Five Element acupuncture diagnosis, the colour white at the sides of the eyes indicates a Metal constitution. This is a shiny, reflective kind of white, not to be confused with the grey, ashen colour that is the lack of red in a person of Fire constitution.

Sound
Weeping

The energy of Metal is a downward movement, so it is natural that the sound of voice that relates to Metal should be one that goes down. Weeping or crying is one of the expressions of sadness, sorrow or grief. While people can also cry from joy or anger, it most usually arises from feelings of loss. It is a normal and natural response to emotional states and yet is commonly suppressed due to parental and cultural influences. Sayings such as 'Big boys don't cry', 'Where's your happy face?' or 'Stop or I'll really give you something to cry about' can lead to a lifetime of emotional suppression.

Cultures vary in the ways that sadness and crying are received and allowed. Men cry far less frequently than women, even though in childhood there is no difference between boys and girls. This suggests that men are expected to suppress their crying. The way people behave at funerals is also illustrative of cultural norms. Some cultures are very reserved in their expression of grief while others are very demonstrative, with loud wailing and sobbing being the norm.

金

Conscious or unconscious suppression of crying will inevitably affect the Metal Element in ways that can have harmful consequences for health, especially the lungs.

The sound of a person's voice is diagnostic of their Constitutional Element. A person of Metal constitution has a weeping voice, one which carries the emotion of grief. What this means is that there is a sound in the voice as if the person were about to burst into tears, even when the topic of conversation is not sad. Many people of Metal constitution have difficulty expressing grief, so the weeping is suppressed in the chest and the sound comes out as a crack or a croak in the voice.

Odour
Rotten

The resonance of odour is the third of the diagnostic tools in determining a person's Constitutional Element. People of a Metal constitution have a subtle odour emanating from their skin which is described, rather unflatteringly, as rotten. When the person is in good health, this odour is faint and light, like the smell of leaves decomposing in autumn. When there is a serious imbalance in the person's health, the odour becomes stronger, resembling that of decaying meat.

The odour arises from the organs of the Element not functioning optimally. In this case, when the large intestine is not eliminating waste in an efficient manner, the body gives off a smell of something rotting.

Emotion

Grief

Since the movement of Metal is downwards, it follows that its emotion will have a falling energy. The overall feeling of the season of autumn is of descent, decay and loss. Loss of warmth, loss of light, loss of growth. The shedding and loss in nature confront the parts of us that have difficulty in letting go of the past. If we are unable to come to terms with the fact that something we cherished is no longer with us, there will be unresolved grief. This may be about a person, a pet, a house, a job, money, a favoured object, even an idea or dream. For many people, the ambient energy of autumn brings subtle reminders of past losses and can reawaken grief about them.

Grief is a normal and natural part of living a human life. In this world where everything that has a beginning also has an end, life becomes studded with many endings. When something we love ends, we are challenged to come to terms with its loss, to honour its place in our life, acknowledge its passing and move on with our life without its presence. The length of time it takes to make this adjustment to loss depends on the depth of its meaning to us. The loss of a parent, child or spouse is clearly going to take much longer to adjust to than the loss of money or possessions. But with all losses, the grief eases with the passage of time.

When there is difficulty in accepting loss, and grief and sadness continue unabated after a long period of time, this becomes damaging to health. So too the suppression of grief affects the health of body and mind. When these emotions are not fully dealt with and processed, they are stored in the lungs and the health of these organs suffers.

For a person of Metal constitution, these issues are primary. Either there is a suppression or denial of grief, or there is an ongoing keening sense of loss. The emotion of grief, feelings of sadness and issues of loss predominate in the Metal person's life.

The organs of Metal are the lungs (yin) and large intestine (yang). From the Western perspective, these are unconnected, but from the perspective of Chinese medicine, they are responsible for letting in and letting out.

Organs and officials

The most important function of the Lung is inhalation. The lungs not only inhale the air and its oxygen, but they also take in the Qi of the air, referred to as Heavenly Qi.[2] If we do not breathe fully and deeply, we are not availing ourselves of this Qi that is freely available to us.

The Lung official is considered to be the principal advisor to the emperor Heart, the Prime Minister who holds the senior role in the government. This is because of Lung's capacity to take in Qi and to regulate its distribution throughout the body in conjunction with the Heart's function of controlling the blood vessels.

The Lung houses the *po*, spirit of Metal. One of the functions of the Lung is to harmonise our spiritual nature with our animal nature, to resolve the conundrum of living as a spiritual being in the body of an animal.

The Large Intestine conducts the waste material from the body, while at the same time reabsorbing water and minerals. Its relationship to Lung is that descending Lung Qi supports the Large Intestine's downward movement; in turn, the Large Intestine Qi helps descending Lung Qi.

At the mental level, the health of the Large Intestine is related to the ability to let go and not dwell upon the past. Hanging on to things that no longer serve, whether this be possessions, thoughts, beliefs or relationships, can be a reflection of Large Intestine imbalance.

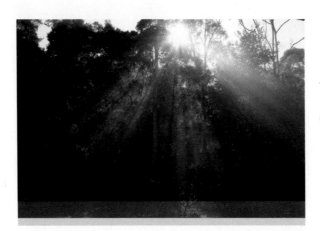

*The breath
of heaven*

We begin our autumnal amble through the points
of the Metal Element by looking at the first point of
the Lung meridian, *Zhongfu* – Middle Palace. Most
acupuncture point location books begin with this
point as the first in the great cycle of all the points.[3]
This is because the ancients believed that when a
newborn takes its first breath in life, the Heavenly
Qi enters the body at this point. It represents the
beginning of life.

    This connection between the Lungs, the breath
and heaven continues throughout our life. With
each breath we take, we inhale not only air but
also Heavenly Qi. It is thought that while most of
our Qi intake is gained through food, 30 per cent
comes from the breath. Middle Palace is a useful
point for helping to open up the chest, making it
easier to collect this free source of energy.

    The *Neijing* states: 'The lung is the advisor [to
the sovereign]. It helps the heart in regulating the
body's Qi.'[4] This Lung official, the senior minister
of the emperor, has the role of overseeing and

Zhongfu
MIDDLE PALACE
Lung 1

regulating the activities of all other ministers. Since Qi is the vital substance that sustains life, and the Lung is responsible for its distribution to all parts of the body, the Lung therefore governs all physiological activity. It controls all the channels through which Qi moves and, in conjunction with the Heart, controls the blood vessels. It also controls ascending and descending Qi as well as the movement of Qi as it enters and exits the meridians.

Zhongfu is both the entry point and the *mu* or alarm point of Lung meridian. As such, it helps with any breathing difficulties such as asthma, coughing, wheezing, nasal congestion and throat obstruction. By opening the chest, it eases chest pain and allows a more upright stance. An open chest helps us to be open to all that the world has to offer us. It supports us to let come what may, to breathe in the world in all its richness.

One of the things that causes congestion at this point is the suppression of emotions. To hold in emotions, there is necessarily a constriction in the breathing. Over time this can produce tightness in the upper chest. Treating *Zhongfu* with either static pressure or vigorous massage can help to loosen such constrictions and let the emotions come forth for expression. Grief is the particular emotion of the Lung and there are sometimes tears stored in this point. It is supportive of those who are grieving.

At the level of spirit, this point can help to reconnect a person with his spiritual nature. It helps him to see the quality and value in his life. It provides access to inspiration, that which is both the taking in of a breath and the divine spark that makes the spirit soar.

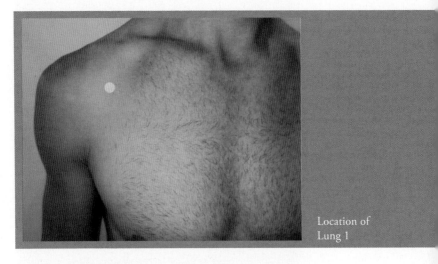

Location of
Lung 1

Lung 1 is located on the outside of the upper chest, 6 cun lateral to the midline and at the level of the first intercostal space. First, find the delto-pectoral triangle, the large hollow directly under the outer third of the collar bone. From here, go down the chest by a thumb's width and move slightly out to the side of the chest. Roll around till you find an area of sensitivity and hold with moderate pressure that is angled towards the midline. Tune in to it as you also pay attention to your breathing. Notice whether there is a change in the sensation, your breathing or your emotions.

Combines with LU 3 · LU 7 · LU 9 · LV 14

Letting go of letting go

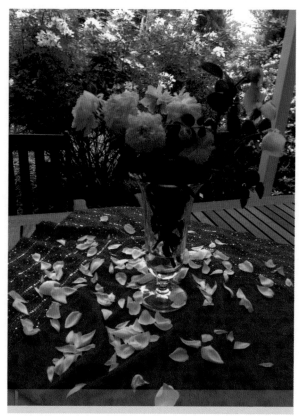

Hegu
JOINING VALLEY
Large Intestine 4

* Forbidden during pregnancy

Years ago I lived in California and met a man who, when he found out I was an acupressure practitioner, told me that was what the police were using to subdue uncooperative suspects. He proceeded to demonstrate, pressing deeply into a point on my hand and another on my arm, points that I know as Large Intestine 4 and 11. The first of these points, *Hegu* – Joining Valley, is certainly an arresting point because of its efficacy in treating a wide range of conditions.

It is probably the best-known acupressure point of all, located in the webbing between the thumb and index finger. Many people know this as good for easing headaches. But this powerful point is also good for constipation, releasing toxins, stress and emotional tension. These are all conditions that involve tightening and hanging on, where there is an inability to let go, relax and be free. This can be a physical holding in the colon or tension in the belly, arms, neck, face and jaw. Or it may be an emotional holding that includes difficulty expressing emotions such as anger and grief, resulting in an inner turmoil.

Letting go of these things is not as simple as it may sound. Friends may advise you, 'Just let go', as if it were as simple as taking off a coat or setting down a suitcase. The problem is that our holding on is not of this kind. Rather, it is borne of long-standing habits, patterns, attitudes and beliefs. Letting go is not something you actually do. In fact, it happens when there is no doing. Letting go is surrender, acceptance. It is being present with what is here now in this moment. Being in the now is the antidote to holding on to memories of the past or projections of the future.

Large Intestine 4 is one of the points of the Metal Element which is at its most obvious in autumn or fall. Autumn teaches us about letting go. Nature is gradually shedding her foliage and daylight hours as she prepares to go within for the winter. This downward-moving energy of Metal supports us in contacting its qualities of acceptance, allowing and surrender.

I invite you to spend some time sitting quietly with this point. By doing so, you will be holding hands with yourself in a quiet, contemplative pose. You will be bringing yourself back to yourself in the present moment. It will support you in letting go of all those things that are no longer helpful to you, no longer in service of your wellbeing.

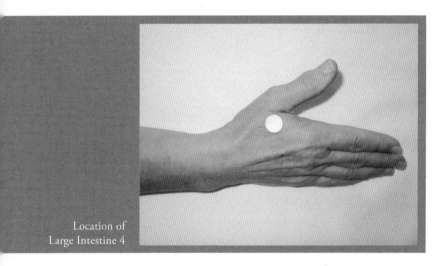

Location of
Large Intestine 4

If you tuck your thumb into the side of your hand, a crease is made. At the end of that crease is a bulge. Press your opposite thumb into the muscle at the highest point of the bulge and direct pressure towards the hand. Roll around until you find a sensitive area. Hold for a few minutes or until the sensitivity decreases. Bring all your attention to the physical sensations and any feelings that may arise.

Combines with LI 11 · LI 15 · LI 18 ·
LU 7 · LU 9 · BL 25 · ST 25 · GB 21

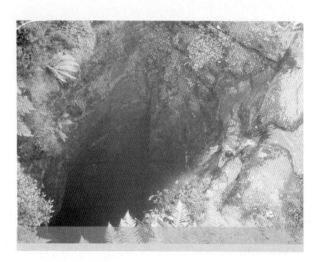

*Catching a breath,
reaching the depth*

In the early years of my practice, I discovered the power of Lung 9 to help asthma sufferers. One client in particular found that by holding this point for herself whenever she felt an asthma attack coming, she was able to reduce the use of her inhalant medication by two-thirds. Lung 9 is the source point of the meridian and, as such, directly relaxes the organ and balances the meridian. Source points are powerful points, and if all you know about acupoints are the 12 source points, you have a valuable set of tools.

Taiyuan
VERY GREAT
ABYSS
Lung 9

Other physical conditions that this point can treat include cough, wheezing, difficult breathing, dry throat, phlegm in the lungs, cold hands, weak voice and the weakness and fragility that result from Qi deficiency.

Later in my practice, I came to discover that Lung 9 can go much deeper, to the psycho-emotional and spiritual levels of a person's being. Indeed, the name of this point, *Taiyuan* – Very

Great Abyss, suggests more profound possibilities than simply treating the lungs.

Very Great Abyss influences the *po* which is the spirit of the Metal Element. Of the five spirits, the *po*, also known as the corporeal soul, is the one that supports the functioning of the body. It is what gives us our instincts and our animal nature. It is our animal soul. Paradoxically, the *po* also allows for that tricky balancing act of living life as a human being, namely that of being a creature of spirit inhabiting the body of an animal.

When the *po* is troubled, this balance between spirit and body, between heaven and earth, can be disturbed. *Taiyuan* is able to go down into the abyss, to the depth of the soul. It can retrieve a person who has lost their way, calm one who is manic and stabilise someone who feels as if they are cracking up or losing control. It can reach down into the very depth of a person, calming, revitalising, rejuvenating and bringing a sense of security and stability.

Whether you simply want to breathe more deeply or if you want to feel more at ease in your body-soul, Very Great Abyss will help bring you back to yourself.

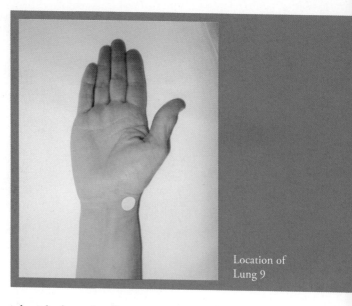

Location of
Lung 9

Hold your hand with the palm facing you. On the radial (thumb) side of the wrist crease, find the hollow between a tendon on the thumb side, the radial artery next to it, and the bone at the base of the hand. Tune into the Qi at the point. Notice how you feel as you hold it. Notice whether it affects your breathing or your mood. If you want to explore further, you can hold it in combination with Large Intestine 4. By holding the two source points of the Metal meridians together, you will be balancing the yin and yang of Metal. Doing this in the autumn, the season of Metal, makes it more powerful still.

Combines with LU 1 · LU 7 · LI 4 · BL 42

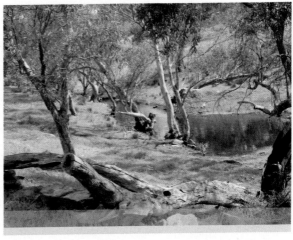

*Anyone for
tennis elbow?*

Quchi
POOL AT THE
CROOK
Large Intestine 11

After the ethereal musings of the first few points of
the Metal Element, we come down to earth with an
examination of a painful physical condition. Tennis
elbow or lateral epicondylitis is a condition that
causes soreness and pain in the outer part of the
elbow. The term 'tennis elbow' is actually a
misnomer; while some cases do derive from playing
the sport improperly, a more likely cause these days
is from the repetitive stress of computer use,
especially mousing. The condition could equally be
called Mouser's Elbow! Half of cases are not even
caused by overexertion but by blows or injuries to
the area.

The acupoint that most effectively addresses
this condition is Large Intestine 11, *Quchi* – Pool
at the Crook. Sustained pressure on this point,
located in the large hollow at the outer end of
the elbow crease, will help to free congested Qi in
this area.

Pool at the Crook has many other uses and can treat a wide range of conditions. As the Earth point of a Metal meridian, it transfers Qi from Earth to Metal and is known as the tonification point of the Large Intestine meridian. It stimulates that organ and is therefore a powerful point for constipation and abdominal congestion. It clears heat from the body and so is useful in cases of fever and inflammation. It can lower blood pressure, relieve toothache and treat pain in the shoulder, upper arm and forearm which lie along the pathway of the meridian.

The skin is the tissue associated with the Metal Element (think of it as a third lung) and so many Metal points are useful for skin problems. *Quchi* is good for treating skin conditions such as eczema, psoriasis and shingles.

Quchi strengthens the Metal Element and can be very grounding for a person who has his head in the clouds. It balances the Qi between Large Intestine and its partner meridian, Lung.

If you or someone you know has elbow pain from a tennis racquet or a mouse, or if they suffer from any of the above ailments, try dipping your finger into the pool at the crook of their elbow.

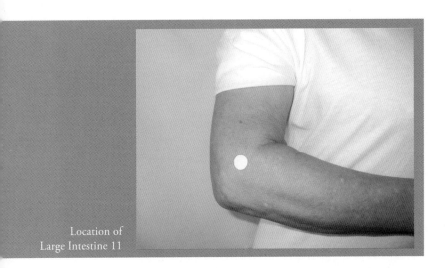

Location of
Large Intestine 11

Place your forearm so that it makes a right angle
with your upper arm, revealing a crease at the outer
edge of the elbow. Place your opposite thumb into
the large hollow at the end of this crease and apply
firm pressure.

Combines with LI 4 · LI 15 · BL 25 · GB 21

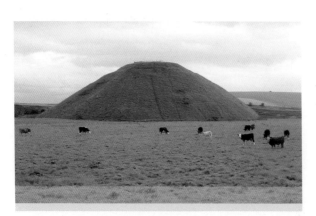

Battle of the bulge

A common problem of the spine is the bulging disc that occurs when the cushioning disc of connective tissue between two vertebrae bulges out, causing inflammation and putting pressure on the nerves that emanate from the spine. A more serious development is a herniated disc which sees a tearing of the outer layer of the disc. Ninety-five percent of spinal disc herniation cases occur in the lower lumbar region at L4 – L5 or L5 – S1.[5] Interestingly, the first of these positions is the location of a point on the Bladder meridian that relates to the Large Intestine.

Dachangshu
LARGE
INTESTINE SHU
Bladder 25

Dachangshu – Large Intestine Shu – can be of great benefit to those suffering from these disc protrusions and other painful conditions of the lumbar region. It is also useful in treating sciatica which originates in the lumbar region and radiates along the pathway of the sciatic nerve, through the buttocks, down the back of the leg and sometimes into the calf and foot.

As the *shu* point of the Large Intestine, *Dachangshu* exerts a strong influence over the organ as well as the functions of the official. When there is stagnation in the intestines, there can be a build-up of waste material resulting in constipation, causing the abdomen to distend and bulge. This in turn creates abdominal discomfort and pain, and sometimes noisy gurgling of the intestines known as borborygmus.

On the other hand, the intestines may be loose, producing loose stools and diarrhoea. When waste moves too quickly through the Large Intestine, water and important minerals cannot be reclaimed and are lost. The Large Intestine *shu* point is helpful in treating conditions at both ends of this constipation–diarrhoea spectrum as well as treating rectal and anal prolapse.

The outer *shu* points are the points that treat the psycho-emotional dimension. As there is no outer *shu* point for the Large Intestine, this inner *shu* point can serve. Where a person is emotionally constipated, holding on to things, people, ideas or beliefs that are no longer of value, or even toxic, *Dachangshu* can assist in the process of letting go. Alternatively, when a person is unable to retain what is valuable and needed to live a healthy life, and lets go of or throws away things and people that are of value, this point is called for.

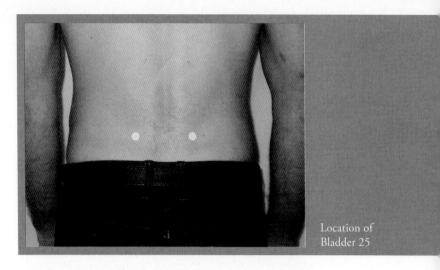

Location of
Bladder 25

Located 1.5 cun lateral to the spine at the level of the junction of the 4th and 5th lumbar vertebrae, the point is tucked into the space above the sacrum and inside the ileum. Apply direct pressure. For treatment of lumbar pain, press both BL 25 points and apply lateral pressure, thereby spreading the tissues of the lower back. This treats the acupoints and releases the fascia of the region.

Combines with LI 4 · LI 11 · ST 25

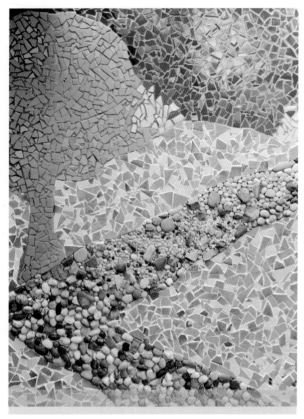

A fork in the road

Lieque
BROKEN
SEQUENCE
Lung 7

It was Yogi Berra who advised: when you come to a fork in the road, take it! The Metal fork we are taking here lies on the pathway of the Lung meridian at the point *Lieque* – Broken Sequence. The break in the sequence refers to the fact that Qi exits the Lung meridian at this point, rather than the last point of the channel, and enters the Large Intestine meridian at LI 4 rather than the first point of that meridian.

The reference to forks doesn't end here. The famous 12th-century physician Ma Danyang, who included this point as one of his Eleven Heavenly Star points, described it as 'a thunderhead splitting fire'.[6] His description is derived from the fact that *Lieque* was an ancient term for lightning which descends to earth in forked bolts. A look at the pathway of Lung channel at this point reveals a sudden deviation that resembles a lightning bolt.

As a significant point on the Lung channel, it treats respiratory conditions such as asthma, phlegmy cough, wheezing and difficult breathing. It is particularly useful for conditions of the nose, including loss of the sense of smell, nasal congestion, discharge and obstruction. Because of its capacity to expel wind, circulate the defensive Qi and stimulate sweating, it is often used in the early stages of colds and flu. For these, its effectiveness is increased when used in combination with LI 4 and LI 20.

Lieque is not only the exit point of Lung, but also the *luo*-connecting point which connects it to the Large Intestine meridian. This twin connection to its partner meridian makes the point doubly effective in treating conditions along the pathway of Large Intestine, including pain and stiffness in the neck, shoulder, throat and face. It also treats constipation and headaches, including migraines.

The emotion of grief is said to reside in the Lung, and *Lieque* is helpful in releasing the oppression of grief and sadness that have been held inside. It helps to open the chest, improve breathing and can facilitate the release of grief by crying.

The influence of this point on Metal is only half of its story, for *Lieque* is also the master point of the *Ren Mai* (Conception Vessel). This vessel is an energy field covering the area from perineum to the chin and which unites all of the yin meridians. *Lieque* can release blocks throughout the Conception Vessel but has a particular effect on the chest, uterus and genitals, and upon a wide range of urinary disorders such as difficult, burning and painful urination.

As the *luo*-connecting point of a yin meridian, it has particular powers to treat psycho-emotional disorders.[7] It assists in letting go of those things that are no longer serving us, making space for the new. It is also known for uncontrolled laughter and frequent yawning. And one final thing before I forget, it is noted especially for poor memory.

So if you forgot where you put that fork, try *Lieque*.

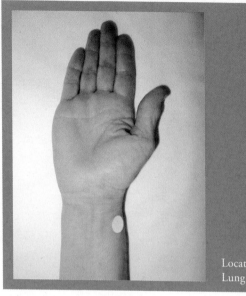

Location of
Lung 7

Located on the side of the radius bone, 1.5 cun
above the wrist crease in a cleft between the tendons
of brachioradialis and abductor pollicis longus. Use
moderate, direct pressure.

Combines with LU 1 · LU 9 · LI 4 ·
LI 20 · CV 17 · K 6

Point of
the shoulder

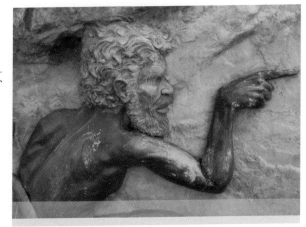

Jianyu
SHOULDER
BONE
Large Intestine 15

The scapula or shoulder blade is a bone that is attached to the rest of the skeleton by one small joint at the point of the shoulder. This is the acromioclavicular (AC) joint. Since this is the only place at which the scapula articulates with the skeleton, a great deal of stress can be placed on this joint.

Otherwise, the scapula is held in place by the 17 muscles that attach to it, connecting it to the arm, chest, ribs, spine and neck in various ways. Given that we all have unique ways of holding and moving our upper body, the positioning of the scapula shows incredibly wide variations among people.

The acupoint that is very close to the AC joint is *Jianyu* – Shoulder Bone – on the Large Intestine meridian. Cross calls this the shoulder chakra, a minor chakra or energy vortex that influences the whole of the shoulder region.[8] It is a powerful point for congestion in the shoulder, since most shoulder problems affect this place where the shoulder meets the arm.

Deadman hails it as the pre-eminent point for treating the shoulder,[9] for it treats paralysis of the arm, shoulder and hand, atrophy of the arm and upper body, arthritis and bursitis of the shoulder, and the chronic condition known as frozen shoulder. It is beneficial when there is an inability to raise the arm to the head, or to turn the head. Overall, it promotes the circulation of Qi and blood throughout the upper arm.

What makes this such a potent point is that, like another important shoulder point SI 10, LI 15 is a meeting point with the Extraordinary Vessel *Yang Qiao Mai* (Yang Motility Vessel) whose trajectory includes the sides of the body from ankle to shoulder, as well as the neck, face and head. Because of this, *Jianyu* releases energy to the brain, provides mental clarity and is good for mental exhaustion and headaches. It works well in conjunction with BL 62 which is the master point of the Yang Motility Vessel.

The point also treats windstroke and clears heat, thereby relieving skin rashes including hives (for which it is best combined with LI 4 and LI 11) and for treating toothache and hypertension. It can control sweating, including underarm perspiration. And it is available as a first aid point for concussion, shock and electric shock.

In short, *Jianyu* helps the shoulder to let go, which reminds us that letting go is one of the functions of the Large Intestine official. Most shoulder tension arises not simply from usage, but from solidified emotional patterns. We hold ourselves in ways that somatically replicate our inner state. Letting go in the shoulder involves letting go of the emotions, ideas and beliefs that dictate our posture and which are no longer of value in our lives.

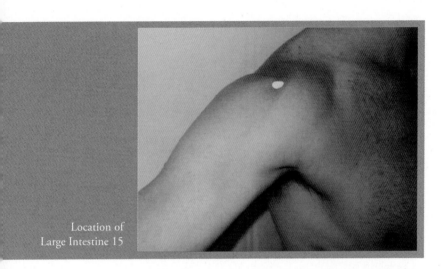

Location of
Large Intestine 15

If you bend your elbow and raise your arm to shoulder height, two hollows appear at the point of the shoulder. LI 15 lies in the anterior (front) hollow. Once located, lower the arm and apply moderate, direct pressure.

Combines with LI 4 · LI 11 ·
LI 18 · BL 62 · SI 10

Smell the roses

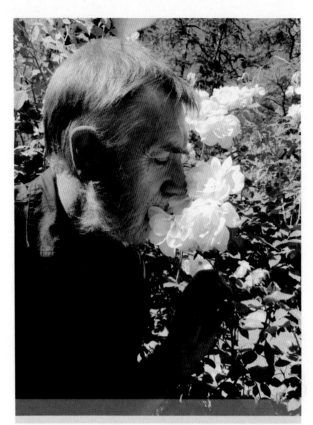

Of all the senses, the sense of smell is the most instinctual, the closest to our animal nature. It is closely connected to survival. It tells us when we are in the presence of something dangerous or toxic such as gas, harmful chemicals or smoke. Smell also helps us to ascertain whether food is good or bad for us, whether it is fresh or has gone off. And it informs us when something or someone is familiar and trusted. Notice how animals use their noses to gather information about all these things.

Yingxiang
WELCOME
FRAGRANCE
Large Intestine 20

When the nose is blocked, not only do we lose the sense of smell, but we can feel somewhat cut off from the world. Breathing becomes more difficult and we are less able to draw in the Heavenly Qi with our breath, less able to breathe in all that life has to offer.

Smell is the sense of the Metal Element. One of the teachings of Metal is to treasure the moment, to be present with all that is here now and to value who you are and what you have. This means breathing in and appreciating the beauty and sweetness of life.

Yingxiang – Welcome Fragrance, the exit point of the Large Intestine meridian, supports us in this endeavour. Fragrance is not simply an odour, but an essence. A healthy Metal distinguishes that which is essential and lets it in.

Qi moves from Welcome Fragrance, the exit point of Large Intestine, to Receiving Tears, the entry point of Stomach meridian. Welcome Fragrance reminds us that Stomach is an Earth meridian and fragrant is the odour of the Earth Element. At the same time, Receiving Tears echoes the grief that is the emotion of the Metal. The connection between Large Intestine and Stomach meridians is a significant one. According to the six channel theory, the two are seen as a single channel called *yangming*. The free flow of Qi between LI 20 and ST 1 (located below the eye) is important. A block here, known as an entry/exit block can produce a serious impediment to treatment.

Yingxiang is the most significant local point for treating all nasal conditions: loss of smell, difficulty breathing, sneezing, nasal congestion and discharge, sinusitis, hay fever, nosebleed and nasal polyps.

It also exerts an influence throughout the face, treating conditions such as red eyes, facial paralysis, tic, trigeminal neuralgia, swelling and itching of the face, pain and swelling in the lips and deviation of the mouth.

Welcome Fragrance invites you to stop for a moment, take time to smell the roses, inhale and appreciate this unique, never-to-be-repeated moment of your life.

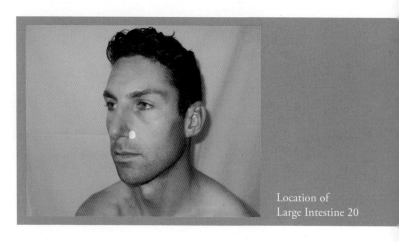

Location of
Large Intestine 20

The point is located in a notch at the side of the nose, at the midpoint of the bulb of the nose. Press towards the sides of the nose. Pressing the points and stretching them away from each other to open the nostrils is also an effective way to treat the points.

Combines with LI 4

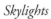

Skylights

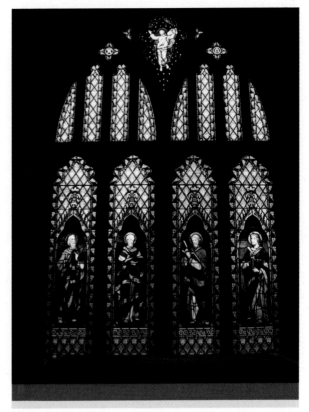

Tianfu
HEAVENLY
PALACE
Lung 3

Futu
SUPPORT AND
RUSH OUT
Large Intestine 18

There is a category of points known as Window of Heaven points, or more commonly Windows of the Sky. Most of these points have in their name the character *tian*, meaning heaven. These points were noted in the *Ling Shu*[10] and by later commentators as useful in treating conditions of the eyes, ears, nose and mouth – the orifices or windows of the head and face. Their function was to reconnect the head (heaven) with the body (earth).

While the classical texts mention no psycho-emotional or spiritual uses of this group, despite the reference to heaven, many modern Five Element practitioners have found that in cases where a person has in some way lost their connection to that which is beyond the physical, these points can indeed be like throwing open the windows of a closed room and letting in the light.

Jarrett believes that window points serve to bring up material from our early life that has been repressed and simultaneously support us in learning from past traumas.[11] For this reason, points should be used later rather than earlier in treatment, and when the person is ready to see and assimilate the truth.

When used from this perspective, these points can bring about significant changes in a person's relationship to the qualities of the Element of the point. In the case of *Tianfu* and *Futu*, they can reconnect a person with the Metal qualities of inspiration, value, purity, respect and surrender.

Tianfu – Heavenly Palace – accesses inspiration, the capacity to be inspired by that which is greater than our small self. Where there is grief and sadness, depression, claustrophobia, agoraphobia, mental confusion, disorientation and forgetfulness that are associated with an imbalance in the Lung official, this point is called for.

When a person suffers from a lack of self-worth, or becomes a perfectionist to compensate for this perception, *Tianfu* can support him in seeing his own value, having self-respect and discovering self-worth. When there is a belief that he is imperfect, and unclean in some way, the point can allow the person to feel cleansed and purified.

Futu – Support and Rush Out – supports the passaging of endings and the letting go of negativity. When a person is stuck in the past, unable to move forward and let go of old beliefs and patterns of behaviour that are no longer working, this point serves. It aids in letting go with the promise that fresher, healthier things will rush into the created space. It clears toxicity from the mind and spirit so that we can reconnect with the influence of heaven and appreciate its value to our life.

Tianfu and *Futu* can usefully be held together as a combination. It is recommended that they also be used in conjunction with their respective source points, Lung 9 and Large Intestine 4. Window points are best used sparingly and approached with reverence. They help us to reconnect with our true nature, the depth of who we are, unalloyed by the structures of the false self.

Recently I was holding *Tianfu* on a client. When I asked her how it felt, she responded with one word: 'Heaven!'

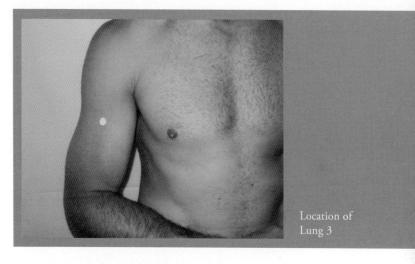

Location of
Lung 3

An interesting classical location is to dab your nose
with ink, then touch your nose to your raised arm
to find the point.[12] More specifically, it is 3 cun
below the crease of the armpit and 6 cun above the
elbow, at the lateral border of the biceps muscle.
If you tense your biceps, the point is found in a
depression between the muscle and the humerus
bone. Use moderate, direct pressure.

Combines with LI 18 · LU 1 · LU 7 · LU 9

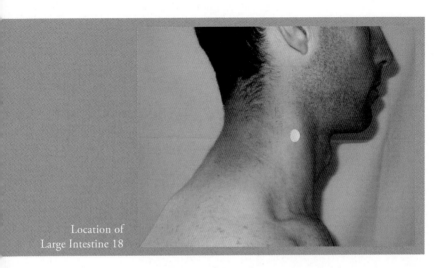

Location of
Large Intestine 18

On the side of the neck, at the level of the Adam's apple, in the space between the two heads of the sternocleidomastoid muscle. This muscle becomes more prominent if the head is turned against resistance to the opposite side. Use gentle, direct pressure.

Combines with LU 3 · LI 4

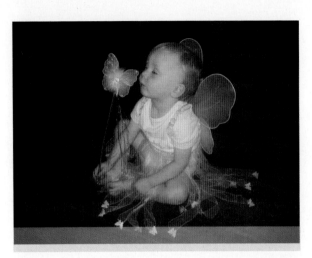

The spirit of Metal

Po is the spirit of the Metal Element. Its character has two parts. The left part is the character for white, which is the colour of the Metal Element.[13] The right part is the character for ghost or earthbound spirit.[14] *Po* is therefore the spirit which is tied to the earth and the mundane.

The *po* is the corporeal soul (sometimes translated as animal soul) which enters the body at conception. In the first months after birth, the baby's whole life revolves around this corporeal soul as it forms the foundation of a healthy body for the life to come. Of the five spirits, it is the only one that disappears when we die. As soon as the lungs exhale for the last time and the body dies, the *po* exits through the anus and descends to join the earth from which it originated.

During life, the *po* is utterly tied to the physical body and to time and space. Like animal instinct, it is concerned with immediate reactions to what is happening in each moment. It is about the here

Pohu
SOUL DOOR
Bladder 42

and the now. This instinctual part of us lives on its senses, alert to all sights, sounds, smells, tastes and textures. It is our animal nature.

The *po* is paired with the *hun*, the ethereal soul which is the spirit of the Wood Element. While the *hun* roams the realm between the earth and the heavens, the *po* provides a counterpoint as the most physical and material part of the human soul. It could be said to be the somatic manifestation of the soul.[15] It provides for clear and sharp sensations and movements and is involved in all physiological processes. Of all these processes, it is especially connected to breathing which is its special province. In fact, the *po* resides in the lungs and is particularly affected by sadness and grief which restrict its movement. Constricted breathing, holding of the breath and shallow breathing are all injurious to the Lung and to the *po*.

While the emotion of grief is the one most closely associated with the *po*, all emotions are ruled by it. It consists of the seven emotions (fear, anxiety, anger, joy, sorrow, worry and grief) which Jarrett neatly describes as 'the primal urges that facilitate the grasping of life'.[16]

Another function of the *po* is to anchor the heavenly aspect of our human nature within the density of the body. It may seem something of a paradox that the spirit which relates so much to our instinctual, animal side is also paramount in connecting us to our spiritual nature. The *po* is concerned with balancing these aspects of our humanness, supporting us as beings of spirit who inhabit the bodies of animals.

Imbalance in the *po* produces a marked disparity between the heavenly and earthly aspects of human life. On the one hand, there can be an obsessive attachment to material things and the accumulation of possessions, money and fame to the detriment of things spiritual. On the other hand, a person may have his head in the clouds and be unable or unwilling to navigate the ordinary world of human existence. There may even be a withdrawal from the world in order to focus on the spiritual search.

Other possible outcomes of *po* imbalance are ongoing physical pain with no identifiable cause, migrating pain, extreme sensitivity to outside psychic influences and chronic health problems associated with emotions that are stuck.[17]

A point that profoundly contacts and balances the *po* is the outer *shu* point of Lung, *Pohu* – Soul Door, sometimes translated as Door of the Corporeal Soul. It is a point that helps to resolve the spirit/animal paradox. It can access the spirit of Metal at a very deep level and serve to reconnect us with what we value in her life, with the preciousness of life itself and with our authentic being or essence. Moreover, it supports us in valuing our essential spiritual nature.

All the longings that we feel are ultimately a desire to be reconnected with spirit, whether or not we are conscious of the underlying nature of our longing. *Pohu* supports reconnection with spirit, and thus can treat all feelings of longing and desire for spirit.

These attributes of *Pohu* are particularly helpful in supporting people in their quest to find spiritual meaning in life on Earth. Where depression, long-term sadness, resignation or lack of inspiration derive from loss of contact with spirit, this soul door offers support.

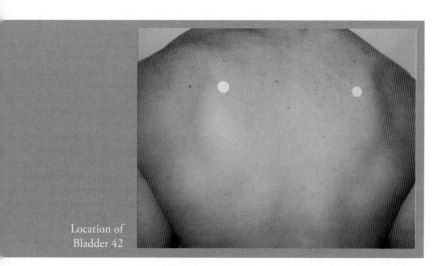

Location of
Bladder 42

The outer *shu* point of the Lung, *Pohu* is located in the upper back, 3 cun lateral to the junction of T3 and T4. The point lies at the medial border of the scapula.

Combines with LU 1 · LU 7 · LU 9

In many temperate climate zones, the transition from autumn to winter is heralded by rain which plucks the final leaves from the deciduous trees. There are still warm days, but it is clear they will not last. Winter is waiting in the wings, ready to roll itself out across the landscape.

For some this can be a difficult transition if it brings with it a foreboding of the chilly days and long cold nights to come, and an unwillingness to let go of the bright days of autumn. For others the transition to winter is welcome, a time to hunker down at home in front of a warm fire with a good book and an early bed, shutting out the world and retreating indoors.

During this transition between autumn and winter, the Metal and Water Elements dance with each other as cold days intersperse themselves in the last of the autumn warmth. We cannot ignore the sun as it dips lower and lower towards the horizon, heading for its rendezvous with the winter solstice. We reach for scarves, vests, extra layers, and think of splitting wood for fires.

Before I began working with the Elements, I hated winter with a passion, dreaded the cold and the dark and the faint depression that descended. But gradually I began to see the rightness of the season, began to accept nature's invitation to go inside. The more we can rest and rejuvenate in this time, the more our internal batteries will be charged in readiness for the next round.

Take up nature's invitation and use this transition period to prepare for turning within. Secure the house against the cold winter winds;

pare back your schedule to allow for early nights; stock up on books, movies, jigsaws, knitting or whatever keeps you comfortable indoors. Emulate the trees and drop the extraneous from your life. Prepare for the descent.

Into yourself.

Going
Further

After delving into the ideas in this book and living with the Elements in their seasons, readers may wish to take the work further. Here are some suggestions.

Journaling

Journaling provides a vehicle for exploring your relationship to each Element in its own season over the course of a year. Keeping a written account of your discoveries is a wonderful way of deepening your experience of the Elements. I recommend buying five journal books in the colours of the Elements: blue, green, red, yellow and white. If you can't find the colours ready to hand, cover the journals with coloured paper. Writing in the green book in spring, for example, brings the vibration of the Wood Element to your writing and keeps it more in your consciousness. You may find that the language you use and even the form and shape of your writing are influenced by the qualities of the Element.

A journal provides a central location for your reflections as you engage with the resonances of each Element. While it is not necessary to write every day, I suggest making regular entries. Even if you feel you have nothing to say, you might begin by inquiring into your reluctance to write about the current season and Element. This can lead to surprising insights.

Entries don't just have to be written. Draw or paint your entries if that is your preferred medium. Cut out images and stick them in. You might even collect materials from nature that reflect the season: leaves, flowers, pollens, twigs, rocks, feathers, insects... The list is yours to complete.

Why is it important to write it all down? Journaling is not simply writing; it is a process of self-reflection, of crystallising thoughts in a way that deepens inquiry. It promotes clarity and honest evaluation that can lead to insight and truth.

Consider your response to the physical conditions of the season: cold, windy, hot, damp, dry. Examine the health of your organs and tissues that relate to each Element and find ways of bringing them to greater health through changes in diet and lifestyle. Note how you react to holding the various acupoints on yourself. Write about how you respond to the psycho-emotional issues presented in the articles. Explore your relationship to the emotion of each Element: fear, anger, joy, sympathy, grief. Investigate the ways in which the spirit of the Element appears in you.

These are just a few suggestions. The blank pages are yours to fill in any way you wish as your relationship with the Elements deepens and unfolds.

Gardening

If you are already a gardener, you will know that this activity keeps you close to nature. By getting your hands in the dirt and making contact with the earth, plants, trees, produce, worms and compost, you stay in touch with the seasons. Over time the gardener learns the rhythms of nature in a profound way. There arises an internal resonance with the external conditions.

Whether you have a big garden with raised beds, a planter box on your patio, or something in between, gardening will keep you close to the qualities of the Elements in ways that support your inner journey around the sheng cycle: through the dormancy and patience of Water, the planning and rapid growth of Wood, the expansion and proliferation of Fire, the satisfaction of Earth's harvest, and the falling away and letting go of Metal.

Hiking

Walking in nature is another great way to connect with the energy of the season and its corresponding Element. Choose a favourite long hike and take the same route in each of the five seasons. Doing the same thing in successive seasons gives you a yardstick by which to chart the changes both in nature and in yourself.

Art

One year I gave myself a little photography project, taking photos of a single tree in each season. It sounds simple, but it required mindfulness to remember to visit the tree five times. In time, the taking of the photographs became secondary to the ritual of connecting with the tree.

Whatever your preferred method of artistic expression, use it as a vehicle to convey your feelings about and your relationship to the Elements. Five drawings. Five paintings. Five sculptures. Five poems. Five songs. Five stories. Five dances.

More acupoints

Want more points? Conduct your own research to find other acupoints, their names, locations, functions and stories about them. Here are some suggestions.

- *Source points.* In this book we looked at all the source points of the yin meridians as well as that of Large Intestine. Check out Stomach 42, Small Intestine 4, Bladder 64, Triple Heater 4 and Gall Bladder 40.

- *Connecting points.* Six are covered in the book. The others are Large Intestine 6, Heart 5, Bladder 58, Kidney 4, Gall Bladder 37 and Liver 5.

- *Shu points.* Six of the outer shu points and two inner shu points were discussed, leaving plenty to choose from among the remaining ten inner and three outer organ shu points.

- *Mu points.* Five of these 'alarm' points are considered in the book. The others are Conception Vessel (CV) 12 (Stomach), Liver 13 (Spleen), CV 14 (Heart), CV 4 (Small Intestine), CV 3 (Bladder), CV 5 (Triple Heater) and Gall Bladder 24 (Gall Bladder).

- *Horary points.* Four of these 'Element of the Element' points were discussed. The others are Lung 8, Large Intestine 1, Heart 8, Small Intestine 5, Bladder 66, Kidney 10, Triple Heater 6 and Liver 1.

- *Tonification points.* These points draw Qi from the mother Element. We investigated three of these. The others are Stomach 41, Spleen 2, Heart 9, Bladder 67, Kidney 7, Heart Protector 9, Triple Heater 3, Gall Bladder 43 and Liver 8. In addition, the yin meridians can be tonified across the *ke* cycle by using the point that corresponds to the Element of the grandmother. These are Kidney 3 (Earth point), Liver 4 (Metal point), Heart 3 (Water point), Heart Protector 3 (Water point), Spleen 1 (Wood point) and Lung 10 (Fire point).

- *Sedation points.* These can be used when the tonification points do not effect the desired Qi transfer. They push Qi from mother to son. It is like taking a stick to the donkey when the carrot of tonification has not worked. These are Lung 5, Large Intestine 2, Stomach 45, Spleen 5, Heart 7, Small Intestine 8, Bladder 65, Kidney 1, Heart Protector 7, Triple Heater 10, Gall Bladder 38 and Liver 2. In addition, the yin meridians can be sedated across the *ke* cycle by using the point that corresponds to the Element of the grandson, namely Kidney 2 (Fire point), Liver 3 (Earth point); Heart 4 (Metal point), Heart Protector 4 (Metal point), Spleen 9 (Water point); and Lung 11 (Wood point).

- *Windows of the Sky.* Light was thrown on four of these. The rest are Stomach 9, Triple Heater 16, CV 22, Small Intestine 16, Small Intestine 17, Heart Protector 1 and Gall Bladder 9.

- *Xi-Cleft or accumulation points.* These points, which were not addressed in this book, can be used to treat acute conditions, i.e. those of sudden onset. They are Lung 6, Large Intestine 7, Stomach 34, Spleen 8, Heart 6, Small Intestine 6, Bladder 63, Kidney 5, Heart Protector 4, Triple Heater 7, Gall Bladder 36 and Liver 6.

- *Entry-exit points.* Where the Qi leaves a meridian of one Element and moves to a meridian of another Element, obstructions in the Qi flow can cause significant blocks to treatment. We looked at several of these. The complete list is Liver 14 – Lung 1;

Large Intestine 20 – Stomach 1; Spleen 21 – Heart 1; Small Intestine 19 – Bladder 1; Kidney 22 – Heart Protector 1; and Triple Heater 22 – Gall Bladder 1.

- *Other important points* not listed above include Large Intestine 10 and 14; Stomach 6, 30 and 37; Spleen 10, 13 and 15; Small Intestine 11; Bladder 6, 7, 40, 53 and 65; Heart Protector 2; Triple Heater 15; Gall Bladder 12, 15, 19 and 39.

Resources

I commend to you the titles in the References and Further Reading lists which follow. For information about the points themselves, I recommend Deadman *et al.* 2005, Dechar 2006, Ellis *et al.* 1989, Hicks 2004, Jarrett 2003 and Kaatz 2005.

To access the wide range of Five Element materials on the internet, I recommend Gye Bennetts' website http://5element.com.au. Gye is an Australian Five Element acupuncturist who has compiled a comprehensive list of internet resources.

Best wishes in your adventure!

Notes

Landscape of the Five Elements

1. Maoshing 1995.
2. Unschuld 1985, pp.252–60.
3. Eckman 1996.
4. Lawson-Wood 1959.
5. Mann 1963.
6. Austin 1972.
7. I have been unable to identify the date on which Worsley began to teach acupuncture. Even Eckman's 1996 brilliant detective work does not pin it down.
8. The four diagnostic tools of colour, sound, odour and emotion (CSOE) are the cornerstone of this method of diagnosis. While there can be a temptation to diagnose by behaviours, CSOE must always form the basis of finding the Constitutional Element.
9. Eckman 1996, p.208, reports observing Worsley identifying the CF of a patient without any of the diagnostic factors, though Eckman declares this was a rare exception.
10. The five notes of the Chinese pentatonic scale are assigned to the Five Elements: La (Water); Mi (Wood); So (Fire); Do (Earth); Re (Metal).
11. Maoshing 1995, p.34.
12. Worsley 1982.
13. Deadman and Khafaji, with Baker 2005.

1. Water

1. Weiger 1965, p.287.
2. Wu 2002, p.87.
3. Deadman et al. 2005, p.340
4. Jarrett 2003, p.416.
5. Jarrett 2003, p.392.
6. Hatton 2000.
7. Maciocia 2005, p.154.
8. M. Buhr, 'Another Way to Think About Qigong's Tricky Gates'. Avaliable at http://internalgongfu. blogspot.co.uk/2014/01/another-way-to-think-about-qigongs.html (accessed 2 July 2005).
9. Newsletters archived at www.acupressure.com.au/newsletter_archive.html.

10. Deadman *et al.* 2005, p.337.
11. Ellis, Wiseman and Boss 1989, p.380.
12. Eckman 1996, p.173.
13. Jarrett 2003, p.452.
14. Jarrett 1998, p.57.
15. Hicks, Hicks and Mole 2004, p.163.
16. Kaptchuk 2000, p.62.
17. Maoshing 1995, p.96.
18. Reninger 2013.

2. Wood

1. Weiger 1965, p.276.
2. Maciocia 2005, p.117.
3. Maciocia 2005, p.200.
4. Deadman *et al.* 2007, p.437.
5. This is Worsley's translation for Liver 14. Its more common name is Cycle Gate since it marks the completion of the whole cycle of the meridian points which begins with Lung 1.
6. Nugent-Head 2012, p.7.
7. Deadman *et al.* 2007, p.447.
8. Ellis *et al.* 1989, p.278.
9. Jarrett 1998, p.236.
10. Dechar 2006, p.199.
11. Wu 2002, p.40.
12. Dechar 2006, p.204.

3. Fire

1. Weiger 1965, p.290.
2. Hicks *et al.* 2004, p.85, notes that speech is the sense organ while the tongue is the orifice. I have taken some liberty here for simplicity.
3. Maciocia 2005, p.71.
4. Larre and Rochat de la Vallee 1992, p.33.
5. Maciocia 2005, p.107.
6. Hicks *et al.* 2004, p.93.
7. Maciocia 2005, p.69.
8. Cross 2006, p.92.
9. Gorman 2011.
10. Wu 2002, p.56.
11. Teeguarden 1978, p.120.
12. Jarrett 2003, p.400.
13. Deadman *et al.* 2007, p.304.

4. Earth

1. Weiger 1965, p.209.
2. Maoshing 1995, p.90.
3. Maoshing 1995, p.116.
4. Barnard 1977, p.434. I find the first two stanzas of Keats' poem 'To Autumn' to be one of the best transmissions of late summer.
5. Hicks *et al.* 2004, p.108.
6. Maoshing 1995, p.21.
7. Veith 1949, p.119.
8. Mann 1963, p.94.
9. Eckman 1996, p.206. I am grateful for Eckman's impeccable scholarship and detective work, which has uncovered this origination.
10. Hicks 2004, p.110.
11. Maciocia 2005, p.185.
12. Unschuld 1986, p.429.
13. Unschuld 1986, p.147.
14. Deadman *et al.* 2007, p.158.
15. Yin, Jin, Qiao *et al.* 2003.
16. Unschuld 1986, p.429.
17. Maoshing 1995, p.47.
18. Kaatz 2005, p.329.
19. Ellis *et al.* 1989, p.103.
20. Deadman *et al.* 2007, p.187.
21. Larre, and Rochat de la Vallee 1997, p.109.
22. Larre and Rochat de la Vallee 1997, p.1.
23. Barnard 1977, p.434.
24. Deadman *et al.* 2007, p.148.
25. Dechar 2006, p.129.
26. Wu 2002, p.65.
27. Weiger 1965, p.187.
28. Maoshing 1995, p.96.
29. Kaptchuk 2000, p.60.
30. Kaptchuk 2000, pp.59–60.
31. Hicks 2004, p.118.

5. Metal

1. Hicks 2004, p.130.
2. Maoshing 1995, p.17.
3. Worsley used Roman numerals to refer to the meridians, beginning with Heart as I and ending with Spleen as XII, a nomenclature adopted by several English acupuncturists. Eckman (1996, p.135) claims this was the result of an error made by Roger de la Fuÿe in transmitting the teachings of George Soulié de Morant.
4. Maoshing 1995, p.34.
5. Moore, Agur and Dalley 2014, p.286.
6. Ellis *et al.* 1989, p.31.
7. Deadman *et al.* 2007, p.85.
8. Cross 2006, p.101.
9. Deadman *et al.* 2007, p.116.
10. Wu 2002, p.99.
11. Jarrett 2003, p.297.
12. Ellis *et al.* 1989, p.26.
13. Weiger 1965, p.223.
14. Weiger 1965, p.112.
15. Maciocia 2005, p.138.
16. Jarrett 1998, p.260.
17. Dechar 2006, p.247.

References

Austin, M. (1972) *Acupuncture Therapy*. New York, NY: ASI Publishers.

Barnard, J. (ed.) (1977) *John Keats: The Complete Poems* (3rd edition). London: Penguin.

Cross, J.R. (2006) *Healing with the Chakra Energy System*. Berkeley, CA: North Atlantic.

Deadman, P. and Ali Khafaji, M., with Baker, K. (2005) *A Manual of Acupuncture* (revised edition). Hove: Journal of Chinese Medicine.

Dechar, L.E. (2006) *Five Spirits*. New York, NY: Lantern.

Eckman, P. (1996) *In the Footsteps of the Yellow Emperor*. San Francisco, CA: Cypress.

Ellis, A., Wiseman, N. and Boss, K. (1989) *Grasping the Wind*. Brookline, MA: Paradigm.

Gorman, J. (2011) 'Scientists hint at why laughter feels so good.' *New York Times*, 13 September. Available at www.nytimes.com/2011/09/14/science/14laughter.html?_r=0, accessed on 23 April 2015.

Hatton, C.L. (ed.) (2000) *Acupuncture Point Compendium*. Leamington: College of Traditional Acupuncture.

Hicks, A., Hicks, J. and Mole, P. (2004) *Five Element Constitutional Acupuncture*. Edinburgh: Churchill Livingstone.

Jarrett, L.S. (1998) *Nourishing Destiny*. Stockbridge, MA: Spirit Path Press.

Jarrett, L.S. (2003) *The Clinical Practice of Chinese Medicine*. Stockbridge, MA: Spirit Path Press.

Kaatz, D. (2005) *Characters of Wisdom*. Soudorgues: Petite Bergerie Press.

Kaptchuk, T.J. (2000) *The Web That Has No Weaver*. Chicago, IL: Contemporary Books.

Larre, C. and Rochat de la Vallee, E. (1992) *The Secret Treatise of the Spiritual Orchid*. Cambridge: Monkey Press.

Larre, C. and Rochat de la Vallee, E. (1997) *The Eight Extraordinary Meridians*. Cambridge: Monkey Press.

Lawson-Wood, D. (1959) *Chinese System of Healing*. Hindhead: Health Sciences Press.

Maciocia, G. (2005) *The Foundations of Chinese Medicine* (2nd edition). Edinburgh: Churchill Livingstone.

Mann, F. (1963) *Acupuncture the Ancient Chinese Art of Healing*. New York, NY: Random House.

Maoshing, N. (trans.) (1995) *The Yellow Emperor's Classic of Medicine*. Boston, MA: Shambala.

Moore, K.L., Agur, A.M.R. and Dalley, A.F. (2014) *Essential Clinical Anatomy* (5th edition). Baltimore, MD: Lippincott Williams & Wilkins.

Nugent-Head, A. (2012) 'The heavenly star points of Ma Danyang.' *Journal of Chinese Medicine 98.*

Reninger, E. (2013) *Wu Wei: The Action of Non-Action.* Available at http://taoism.about.com/od/wuwei/a/wuwei.htm, accessed on 24 April 2015.

Teeguarden, I.M. (1978) *Acupressure Way of Health.* Tokyo: Japan.

Unschuld, P.U. (1985) *Medicine in China.* Berkeley, CA: UC Press.

Unschuld, P.U. (trans.) (1985) *Nan-ching: The Classic of Difficulties.* Berkeley, CA: UC Press.

Veith I. (trans.) (1949), *The Yellow Emperor's Classic of Internal Medicine.* Baltimore, MD: Williams & Wilkins.

Weiger, L. (1965) *Chinese Characters.* New York, NY: Dover.

Worsley, J.R. (1982) *Traditional Chinese Acupuncture Volume 1 Meridians and Points.* Tisbury: Element Books.

Wu, J.N. (2002) *Ling Shu or the Spiritual Pivot.* Honolulu, HI: University of Hawaii Press.

Yin, L., Jin, X., Qiao, W. *et al.* (2003) 'PET imaging of brain function while puncturing the acupoint ST36.' *Chinese Medical Journal 116,* 12, 1836–1839.

Further Reading

Beinfield, H. and Korngold, E. (1991) *Between Heaven and Earth*. New York, NY: Ballantine.

Connelly, D.M. (1994) *Traditional Acupuncture: The Law of the Five Elements* (2nd edition). Columbia, MD: Traditional Acupuncture Institute.

Cross, J.R. (2008) *Acupuncture and the Chakra Energy System*. Berkeley, CA: North Atlantic.

Dolowich, G. (2003) *Archetypal Acupuncture: Healing with the Five Elements*. Aptos, CA: Jade Mountain.

Fung, Y.L. (1976) *A Short History of Chinese Philosophy*. New York, NY: Free Press. (Original work published in 1949.)

Gach, M.R. (2004) *Acupressure for Emotional Healing*. New York, NY: Bantam.

Haas, E.M. (1981) *Staying Healthy with the Seasons*. Berkeley, CA: Celestial Arts.

Hammer, L. (1990) *Dragon Rises, Red Bird Flies*. Seattle, WA: Eastland.

Hicks, A. and Hicks, J. (1999) *Healing Your Emotions*. London: Thorsons.

Jarmey, C. and Bouratinos, I. (2008) *A Practical Guide to Acupoints*. Berkeley, CA: North Atlantic.

Larre, C. and Rochat de la Vallee, E. (1995) *Rooted in Spirit*. Barrytown, NY: Station Hill.

Maciocia, G. (2009) *The Psyche in Chinese Medicine*. Edinburgh: Churchill Livingstone.

Marin, G. (2006) *Five Elements Six Conditions*. Berkeley, CA: North Atlantic.

Matsumoto, K. and Birch, S. (1986) *Extraordinary Vessels*. Brookline, MA: Paradigm.

Mitchell, S. (1988) *Tao Te Ching*. New York, NY: Harper.

Moss, C.A. (2010) *Power of the Five Elements*. Berkeley, CA: North Atlantic.

Reichstein, G. (1998) *Wood Becomes Water*. New York, NY: Kodansha.

Teeguarden, I.M. (1987) *The Joy of Feeling*. Tokyo: Japan Publications.

Teeguarden, I.M. (1996) *A Complete Guide to Acupressure*. Tokyo: Japan Publications.

Acknowledgements

These acknowledgements could be regarded as a continuation of the chapter on the Metal Element, whose gifts include recognition, reverence, appreciation and respect. With all of these qualities in mind, I bow to the many people who have supported the evolution of this book.

Acknowledgements are due to all of my teachers on the Five Element path, including Geoff Marshall, Iona Teeguarden, Michael Berry, Dianne Connelly, Bob Duggan, Julia Measures, John Sullivan, J.R. Worsley and Judy Worsley. Fond thanks to my fellow members of Five Hands Clapping, Tom Balles, Devi Brown, Jenny Josephian, Susan Leahy, Daniel Meyerovich and Keith Stetson. The work we did together in the '90s shaped the platform for this book. Also my respect to the many authors of books on Five Element acupuncture and Chinese medicine whose works have inspired me.

Many thanks to Persephone Maywald whose painstaking editing of my early newsletters taught me how to write. Gratitude to my good friend Lisa Fabry for her gentle editing of *Seasons of Life*, the soon to be published precursor to this work. Hat off to Peter Farnsworth for his ongoing support of my work and for putting me on to Singing Dragon Publishers. Thanks also to Tony Fonseka for his reading and helpful comments, and to the many friends, clients and students, too numerous to mention, who have given me such positive support in the writing process.

Thanks to Steve Davis of Baker Marketing for showing me the importance of blogging, and to Sam Barakat for providing the timely kick in the pants that got me started. And to Jessica Kingsley for seeing the potential in my blog and really understanding about living with the Five Elements.

Appreciation to Lorie Dechar and Gail Rex-Reichstein for their kind willingness to review this book and for their generous endorsements.

To my Kirkwood family members Barb, Ken, Peter, Mardi, Tia and Eve for their love and support.

Loving thanks to Margaret Towie for helping me to open my heart, allowing love to flavour the words I write.

With great love and gratitude to Hameed Ali whose teachings have shown me the path of runaway realisation. To my Diamond Approach teachers Karen Johnson, Vince Draddy, Sarah Stanke, Laurie Wattel and Lauren Armstrong; and all my Diamond Heart friends and inquiry partners including Jackie Marlu, J.R. Miller, Diana Clarke, Kimberley Lemyre, Ann Fitts, B. Vohryzek and Steve March. Heartfelt thanks to Vince for his seminal question, 'What about the book?' and his 15 years of support for being who I truly am.

And most importantly of all, my profound love and gratitude to true nature, the nature of me, you and everything. When I remember that it isn't me who is doing the writing, I can watch on with delight as writing arises from the void.

Index